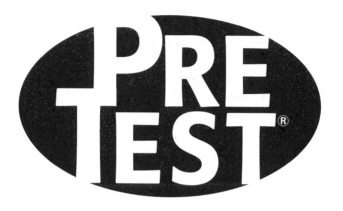

Preventive Medicine and Public Health

PreTest® Self-Assessment and Review

Notice

Medicine is an ever-changing science. As new research and clinical experience broaden our knowledge, changes in treatment and drug therapy are required. The authors and the publisher of this work have checked with sources believed to be reliable in their efforts to provide information that is complete and generally in accord with the standards accepted at the time of publication. However, in view of the possibility of human error or changes in medical sciences, neither the authors nor the publisher nor any other party who has been involved in the preparation or publication of this work warrants that the information contained herein is in every respect accurate or complete, and they disclaim all responsibility for any errors or omissions or for the results obtained from use of the information contained in this work. Readers are encouraged to confirm the information contained herein with other sources. For example and in particular, readers are advised to check the product information sheet included in the package of each drug they plan to administer to be certain that the information contained in this work is accurate and that changes have not been made in the recommended dose or in the contraindications for administration. This recommendation is of particular importance in connection with new or infrequently used drugs.

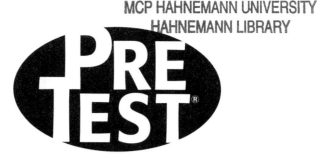

Preventive Medicine and Public Health

PreTest® Self-Assessment and Review

Ninth Edition

SYLVIE RATELLE, M.D., M.P.H.

Director
STD/HIV Prevention Training Center of New England
Medical Consultant
Division of Sexually Transmitted Diseases Prevention
Massachusetts Department of Public Health, Boston, Massachusetts
Assistant Professor
Department of Family and Community Medicine
Associate Director, Preventive Medicine Residency Program
University of Massachusetts School of Medicine, Worcester, Massachusetts

STUDENT REVIEWERS

NATALIE F. HOLT

Yale University School of Medicine, New Haven, Connecticut

LUCY CHIE

MEGAN SCHWARZMAN

University of Massachusetts School of Medicine, Worcester, Massachusetts

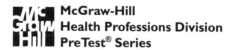 **McGraw-Hill**
Health Professions Division
PreTest® Series

NEW YORK ST. LOUIS SAN FRANCISCO AUCKLAND
BOGOTÁ CARACAS LISBON LONDON MADRID
MEXICO CITY MILAN MONTREAL NEW DELHI
SAN JUAN SINGAPORE SYDNEY TOKYO TORONTO

McGraw-Hill

A Division of The **McGraw·Hill** Companies

Preventive Medicine and Public Health: PreTest Self-Assessment and Review, Ninth Edition

Copyright © 2001, 1998, 1995, 1992, 1989, 1987, 1985, 1980, 1976 by the **McGraw-Hill Companies**, Inc. All rights reserved. Printed in the United States of America. Except as permitted under the United States Copyright Act of 1976, no part of this publication may be reproduced or distributed in any form or by any means, or stored in a data base or retrieval system, without the prior written permission of the publisher.

1 2 3 4 5 6 7 8 9 0 DOC/DOC 0 9 8 7 6 5 4 3 2 1

WA 18.2 P9445 2000

ISBN 0-07-135962-1

This book was set in Berkeley by North Market Street Graphics.
The editor was Catherine Wenz.
The production supervisor was Rohnda Barnes.
Project management was provided by North Market Street Graphics.
The text designer was Jim Sullivan / RepCat Graphics & Editorial Services.
The cover designer was Li Chen Chang / Pinpoint.
R.R. Donnelley & Sons was printer and binder.

This book is printed on acid-free paper.

Library of Congress Cataloging-in-Publication Data

Preventive medicine and public health : PreTest self-assessment and review / editor, Sylvie Ratelle—9th ed.
    p. ; cm.
  Includes bibliographical references.
  ISBN 0-07-135962-1 (pbk.)
   1. Public health—Examinations, questions, etc. 2. Medicine, Preventive—Examinations, questions, etc. 3. Epidemiology—Examinations, questions, etc. I. Ratelle, Sylvie.
  [DNLM: 1. Public Health—Examination Questions. 2. Epidemiology—Examination Questions. 3. Preventive Medicine—Examination Questions. WA 18.2 P944 2000]
RA430 .P74 2000
614.4'076—dc21   00-041564

CONTENTS

PREFACE

Many changes have been made in this book from the last edition. I hope it will be helpful in providing a good review of public health and preventive medicine. I also hope you will appreciate how applicable this field is in everyday clinical practice (even biostatistics principles!) and what an important impact prevention can have on the health of a population. Many thanks to the medical students, Lucy Chie, Megan Schwarzman, and Natalie Holt, for their thoughtful comments.

This book is dedicated to my husband, Alain Campbell, M.D., M.S., and my daughter, Myriam. Very special thanks for supporting me throughout this project.

SYLVIE RATELLE, M.D., M.P.H.

INTRODUCTION

Preventive Medicine and Public Health: PreTest® Self-Assessment and Review, Ninth Edition, has been designed to provide medical students and physicians with a comprehensive and convenient instrument for self-assessment and review within the field of epidemiology and public health. The 500 questions provided have been designed to parallel the format of the questions contained in Step 2 of the United States Medical Licensing Examination (USMLE).

Each question in the book is accompanied by an answer, a paragraph explanation, and a specific page reference to either a current journal article, a textbook, or both. A bibliography that lists all the sources used in the book follows the last chapter.

Perhaps the most effective way to use this book is to allow yourself one minute to answer each question in a given chapter; as you proceed, indicate your answer beside each question. By following this suggestion, you will be approximating the time limits imposed by licensing examinations.

When you practice your examination-taking skills with this PreTest®, one way to maximize your score is to go through, answer all the questions you find easy, and skip over the more difficult ones initially. We do recommend, however, that once you come back to the more difficult questions, you spend as much time as you need. You will then be more likely to retain the information. *Do note:* When it comes to your examination for the board, you will do better to answer each question as you come to it and not skip around. Do not spend too much time on any one problem. Make a guess, circle the question, and come back to it. Otherwise, you can waste time looking for the questions you skipped or—the ultimate tragedy—you may discover time is running out.

When you have finished answering the questions in a chapter, you should then spend as much time as you need verifying your answers and carefully reading the explanations. Although you should pay special attention to the explanations for the questions you answered incorrectly, you should read every explanation. The author of this book has designed the explanations to reinforce and supplement the information tested by the questions. If, after reading the explanations for a given chapter, you feel you need still more information about the material covered, you may wish to consult the references indicated.

BIOSTATISTICS AND METHODS OF EPIDEMIOLOGY

Questions

DIRECTIONS: Each item below contains a question or incomplete statement followed by suggested responses. Select the **one best** response to each question.

1. Assuming that mammography has a sensitivity of 90% and a specificity of 98% and that consecutive tests are independent, what is the probability that a woman with breast cancer will have a negative yearly screening mammogram for two consecutive years?

a. 1/10
b. 2/10
c. 4/10
d. 1/100
e. 4/100

2. The association between low birth weight and maternal smoking during pregnancy can be studied by obtaining smoking histories from women at the time of the first prenatal visit and then subsequently assessing and assigning birth weight at delivery according to smoking histories. What type of study is this?

a. Clinical trial
b. Cross-sectional
c. Prospective cohort
d. Case-control
e. Retrospective cohort

3. An investigator wishes to perform a randomized clinical trial to evaluate a new beta blocker as a treatment for hypertension. To be eligible for the study, subjects must have a resting diastolic blood pressure of at least 90 mm Hg. One hundred patients seen at the screening clinic with this level of hypertension are recruited for the study and make appointments with the study nurse. When the nurse obtains their blood pressure two weeks later, only 65 of them have diastolic blood pressures of 90 mm Hg or more. The most likely explanation for this is

a. Spontaneous resolution
b. Regression toward the mean
c. Baseline drift
d. Measurement error
e. Hawthorne effect

4. Which of the following measures is used frequently as a denominator to calculate the incidence rate of a disease?

a. Number of cases observed
b. Number of new cases observed
c. Number of asymptomatic cases
d. Person-years of observation
e. Persons lost to follow-up

5. Among women aged 18 to 34 in a community, weight is normally distributed with a mean of 52 kg and a standard deviation of 7.5 kg. What percentage of women will have a weight over 59.5 kg?

a. 2%
b. 5%
c. 10%
d. 16%
e. 32%

6. In nine families surveyed, the numbers of children per family were 4, 6, 2, 2, 4, 3, 2, 1, and 7. The mean, median, and mode numbers of children per family are, respectively,

a. 3.4, 2, 3
b. 3, 3.4, 2
c. 3, 3, 2
d. 2, 3.5, 3
e. 3.4, 3, 2

7. A study is undertaken to determine whether drinking more than eight cups of coffee a day is associated with hypertension. The blood pressure readings were taken of persons who drink more than eight cups and persons who drink no coffee. The results are as follows:

	Hypertension	Normal Blood Pressure	Total
>8 cups	6	4	10
No coffee	2	7	9
	8	11	19

Which of the following is the most appropriate test to analyze the data?

a. Chi-square test
b. McNemar's test
c. Fisher's exact test
d. Student t test
e. Analysis of variance

Items 8–10

The results of a study of the incidence of pulmonary tuberculosis in a village in India are given in the following table. All persons in the village are examined during two surveys made two years apart, and the number of new cases was used to determine the incidence rate.

Category of Household at First Survey	Number of Persons	Number of New Cases
With culture-positive case	500	10
Without culture-positive case	10,000	10

8. What is the incidence of new cases per 1000 person-years in households that had a culture-positive case during the first survey?

a. 0.02
b. 0.01
c. 1.0
d. 10
e. 20

9. What is the incidence of new cases per 1000 person-years in households that did not have a culture-positive case during the first survey?

a. 0.001
b. 0.1
c. 0.5
d. 1.0
e. 5.0

10. What is the relative risk of acquiring tuberculosis in households with a culture-positive case compared with households without tuberculosis?

a. 0.05
b. 0.5
c. 2.0
d. 10
e. 20

11. In the study of the cause of a disease, the essential difference between an experimental study and an observational study is that in the experimental investigation

a. The study is prospective
b. The study is retrospective
c. The study and control groups are of equal size
d. The study and control groups are selected on the basis of history of exposure to the suspected causal factor
e. The investigators determine who is and who is not exposed to the suspected causal factor

Items 12–13

About 1% of boys are born with undescended testes. To determine whether prenatal exposure to tobacco smoke is a cause of undescended testes in newborns, the mothers of 100 newborns with undescended testes and those of 100 newborns whose testes had descended were questioned about smoking habits during pregnancy. The study revealed an odds ratio of 2.6 associated with exposure to smoke, with 95% confidence intervals (CI) from 1.1 to 5.3.

12. Some reviewers are concerned that the study may overestimate the association between maternal smoking and undescended testes in the offspring because of potential

a. Confounding
b. Nondifferential misclassification
c. Differential misclassification
d. Selection bias
e. Loss to follow-up

13. What is the most appropriate conclusion to be drawn from the study?

a. There is no association between maternal smoking and undescended testes in the offspring
b. The study results, if accurate, suggest that an offspring whose mother smoked is about 2.6 times more likely to be born with undescended testes than an offspring whose mother did not smoke
c. The p value > 0.05
d. The 90% confidence interval for these results would probably include 1.0
e. A larger sample size would increase the confidence interval

14. The probability of being born with condition A is 0.10 and the probability of being born with condition B is 0.50. If conditions A and B are independent, what is the probability of being born with either condition A or condition B (or both)?

a. 0.05
b. 0.40
c. 0.50
d. 0.55
e. 0.60

15. As an epidemiologist, you are asked to recommend the type of study appropriate to the needs of researchers who would like to study the causes of a rare form of sarcoma. They have discovered a registry of this form of cancer and have access to the largest database of patients with this form of cancer, which, unfortunately, is only a few years old. They have funding for only one year from the National Institutes of Health and note the budget will be tight. What type of study design do you recommend?

a. Prospective cohort
b. Retrospective cohort
c. Cross-sectional
d. Experimental
e. Case-control

16. If rapidly progressive cancers are missed by a screening test, which type of bias will occur?

a. Lead-time bias
b. Length bias
c. Selection bias
d. Surveillance bias
e. Information bias

Items 17–19

Lou Stewells, a pioneer in the study of diarrheal disease, has developed a new diagnostic test for cholera. When his agent is added to the stool, the organisms develop a characteristic ring around them. (He calls it the "Ring-Around-the-Cholera" [RAC] test.) He performs the test on 100 patients known to have cholera and 100 patients known not to have cholera with the following results:

	Cholera	No Cholera
RAC test +	91	12
RAC test −	9	88
Totals	100	100

17. Which of the following statements is INCORRECT about the RAC test?

a. The sensitivity of the test was about 91%
b. The specificity of the test was about 12%
c. The false negative rate was about 9%
d. The predictive value of a positive result cannot be determined from the preceding information
e. The predictive value of a negative result cannot be determined from the preceding information

18. Dr. Stewells next performs the test on 1000 patients with profuse diarrhea:

	Cholera	No Cholera
RAC test +	312	79
RAC test −	31	578
Totals	343	657

Which of the following statements is correct?

a. The predictive value of a positive result is 31/343
b. The predictive value of a positive result is 79/312
c. The predictive value of a negative result is 578/(578 + 31)
d. The predictive value of a negative test is 578/657
e. The incidence rate of cholera in this population is 343/1000

19. The RAC test achieves widespread acceptance. However, with improvements in hygiene, the prevalence of cholera gradually falls from 35 to 5% of hospitalized diarrhea patients. Which statement about the effect of this fall in prevalence is true?

a. The change in prevalence will reduce the predictive value of a negative result
b. The predictive value of a positive result will decline
c. The specificity of the test is likely to decline
d. The specificity of the test will increase at the expense of its sensitivity
e. It will have no impact on the predictive values of the test

20. A randomized clinical trial is undertaken to examine the effect of a new combination of antiretroviral drugs on HIV viral load compared to usual therapy. Randomization is used for allocation of subjects to either treatment or control (usual care) groups in experimental studies. Randomization ensures that

a. Assignment occurs by chance
b. Treatment and control (usual care) groups are alike in all respects except treatment
c. Bias in observations is eliminated
d. Placebo effects are eliminated
e. An equal number of persons will be followed in the treatment and control group

21. In a study of the cause of lung cancer, patients who had the disease were matched with controls by age, sex, place of residence, and social class. The frequency of cigarette smoking was then compared in the two groups. What type of study was this?

a. Prospective cohort
b. Retrospective cohort
c. Clinical trial
d. Case-control
e. Correlation

Items 22–24

The incidence rate of lung cancer is 120/100,000 person-years for smokers and 10/100,000 person-years for nonsmokers. The prevalence of smoking is 20% in the community.

22. What is the relative risk of developing lung cancer for smokers compared with nonsmokers?

a. 5
b. 12
c. 50
d. 100
e. 120

23. What percentage of lung cancer can be attributed to smoking?

a. 52%
b. 78%
c. 80%
d. 92%
e. 99%

24. If the prevalence of smoking in the community was decreased to 10%, the excess incidence rate of lung cancer that could be averted in that community would be

a. 11/100,000
b. 22/100,000
c. 50/100,000
d. 60/100,000
e. 110/100,000

25. The Coronary Drug Project was a randomized trial to evaluate the efficacy of several lipid-lowering drugs. The five-year mortality of the men who adhered to the regimen of clofibrate (i.e., took 80% of their medicine or more) was 15%; among those assigned to the clofibrate group who were less compliant, it was 24.6%. The result was highly statistically significant ($p < 0.0001$). From this one can conclude

a. Clofibrate was very beneficial to the patients who took it reliably
b. Clofibrate is not effective unless patients take at least 80% of the recommended doses
c. Either clofibrate or something associated with taking it reliably is strongly associated with reduced total mortality
d. There was a problem with blinding in this study
e. Only those who were compliant should be included in the data

26. The use of matching as a technique to control for confounding is most appropriate for which type of study?

a. A large-scale cohort study
b. A case-control study with a small number of cases
c. A clinical trial with a factorial design
d. A cross-sectional study with multiple variables
e. A correlation study with a small number of countries

Items 27–28

An investigator is designing a randomized, double-blind, placebo-controlled clinical trial to see whether vitamin E will prevent lung cancer.

27. Which technique is likely to maximize compliance with the allocated regimen?

a. Using the placebo
b. Performing a run-in phase
c. Using intent-to-treat analysis
d. Double blinding the study
e. Limiting the number of subjects enrolled

28. Which is most likely to affect the validity (source of bias) of the study?

a. Loss to follow-up
b. Incidence of lung cancer
c. Prevalence of smoking in the source population
d. α error
e. β error

29. The crude death rate in the United States is 150/100,000. The crude death rate in a smaller, developing country is 75/100,000. Based on these data, which one of the following statements best explains the data?

a. The health care system of the developing country is far better than that in the United States
b. More people die in the United States because it has a larger population
c. Infant mortality in the first week is higher in developing countries, but it is not included in the crude death rate
d. Death rates in the developing country are lower due to the emigration effect
e. Crude death rates are usually higher in developed countries because of a higher proportion of older persons in the population

Items 30–32

A research team wishes to investigate a possible association between smokeless tobacco and oral lesions among professional baseball players. At spring training camp, they ask each baseball player about current and past use of smokeless tobacco, cigarettes, and alcohol, and a dentist notes the type and extent of the lesions in the mouth.

30. What type of study is this?

a. Case-control
b. Cross-sectional
c. Prospective cohort
d. Clinical trial
e. Retrospective cohort

31. After the players have been questioned about use of smokeless tobacco and examined for lesions of the mouth, the data on the 146 players are tabulated as follows:

	Mouth Lesion	No Lesion	Total
User	80	30	110
Nonuser	2	34	36
Total	82	64	146

In this study, which measure of disease occurrence can be calculated?
a. Incidence rate
b. Cumulative incidence rate
c. Incidence density
d. Prevalence
e. Relative risk

32. Which of the following statements is true?
a. The odds ratio is equal to $(80/110) \times (2/36) = 13.1$
b. A temporal association between smokeless tobacco use and oral lesions can be established
c. The statistical association can be calculated using the chi-square test
d. Selection bias could overestimate the result
e. There should be an equal number of exposed and nonexposed subjects

33. A randomized trial shows that a new thrombolytic agent reduces total mortality by 30% in the first 30 days after a suspected myocardial infarction compared with a placebo ($p = 0.002$). Which of the following questions would be the most important to have answered?
a. Was the trial blinded?
b. What was the power of the study?
c. What happened to surviving patients in the next year?
d. What percentage of patients in each group actually had a myocardial infarction?
e. What was the effect on mortality from coronary heart disease?

Items 34–36

In a study of the effectiveness of pertussis vaccine in preventing pertussis (whooping cough), the following data were collected by studying siblings of children who had the disease.

Immunization Status of Sibling Contact	Number of Siblings Exposed to Case	Number of Cases among Siblings
Complete	4000	400
None	1000	400

34. What was the secondary attack rate of pertussis in fully immunized household contacts?

a. 0%
b. 10%
c. 25%
d. 40%
e. 75%

35. What was the protective efficacy of whooping cough vaccine?

a. 25%
b. 40%
c. 75%
d. 90%
e. 99%

36. What was the relative risk of contracting whooping cough in the unimmunized children compared with the fully immunized children?

a. 0.25
b. 0.5
c. 1.0
d. 2.0
e. 4.0

37. Decision analyses often include a patient's utilities in the determination of the best decision. These utilities measure

a. Whether a patient favors one decision over another
b. Whether a physician favors one decision over another
c. The difference between a patient's decision and the physician's decision
d. The relative value a patient places on a particular outcome
e. The relative likelihood of a particular outcome

38. You have just finished conducting a case-control study to measure the association between alcohol use and lower respiratory tract infections. The most appropriate method to control for smoking as a confounder is

a. Matching
b. Restriction
c. Randomization
d. Stratification
e. Multivariate modeling

Items 39–41

Data from an investigation of an epidemic of rubella in a remote village in Brazil are given in the following table:

Age Group (years)	Number in Population	Number Ill (Symptomatic)	Number Not Ill but with Antibody Rise (Asymptomatic)	Number Uninfected	Percent Infected
0–9	204	110	74	20	90
10–19	129	70	46	13	90
20–39	161	88	57	16	90
40–59	78	42	28	8	90
60+	42	2	2	38	10
Totals	614	312	207	95	

39. Which expression represents the calculation to determine the incidence of illness (symptomatic cases) for all age groups (as a percentage)?

a. $95/519 \times 100\% = 18.3\%$
b. $207/614 \times 100\% = 33.7\%$
c. $207/519 \times 100\% = 39.9\%$
d. $312/614 \times 100\% = 50.8\%$
e. $519/614 \times 100\% = 84.5\%$

40. Which expression represents the calculation to determine the percentage of infection that is asymptomatic (subclinical)?

a. $95/519 \times 100\% = 18.3\%$
b. $207/614 \times 100\% = 33.7\%$
c. $207/519 \times 100\% = 39.9\%$
d. $312/614 \times 100\% = 50.8\%$
e. $519/614 \times 100\% = 84.5\%$

41. Based on the age-specific infection rates, when did German measles previously occur in this village in relation to the current epidemic?

a. 0 to 9 years ago
b. 10 to 19 years ago
c. 20 to 39 years ago
d. 40 to 59 years ago
e. 60 or more years ago

Items 42–44

A new test has been developed to screen for ovarian cancer. The following figure illustrates the distribution of values for this test among two populations.

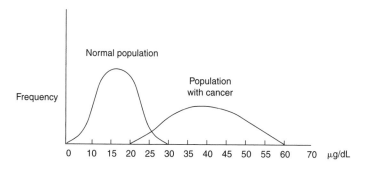

42. If the researcher chooses values under 30 μg/dL as normal limits for the test, which of the following statements is true?

a. The test will be 100% specific
b. The test will be 100% sensitive
c. Some persons without cancer will test positive
d. There will be some false-positive tests
e. All persons with cancer will have a positive test

43. If the researcher chooses values under 25 μg/dL as normal limits for the test, which of the following statements is true?

a. The test will be 100% specific
b. The test will be 100% sensitive
c. No false-negative tests will occur
d. There will be some false-positive tests
e. All persons with cancer will have a positive test

44. The researcher decides to use values under 20 μg/dL as normal limits, and the test becomes commercially available. One of your patients has a test result of 27 μg/dL. You conclude that

a. The patient has cancer of the ovary
b. The patient does not have cancer of the ovary
c. This is a false-negative test
d. A confirmation test will be needed as she may or may not have cancer
e. This test is not sensitive enough to detect cancer

45. You are preparing a report to present to the Public Health Council on the declining rates of gonorrhea in your state in both men and women over the last 10 years. Which type of graph would best illustrate the data?

a. Bar chart
b. Histogram
c. Pie chart
d. Frequency polygon
e. Line graph

46. Consider the following two distribution curves.

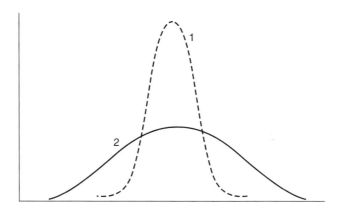

Which numerical summary measure would allow you to discriminate between the two distributions?

a. Median
b. Mean
c. Mode
d. Standard deviation
e. Sample size

47. Consider the following distribution curve.

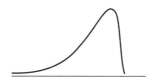

Which statement best applies to this curve?

a. The mean is a more robust measure of central tendency
b. The median is larger than the mean
c. The data is skewed to the right
d. This is a normal distribution
e. This is a bimodal distribution

Items 48–50

Five prospective cohort studies were undertaken to examine the association between bacterial vaginosis and delivery of a premature child. The results of these five hypothetical studies are illustrated in the following figure and are expressed as relative risks with 95% confidence intervals.

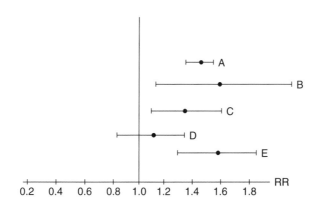

48. Which study appears to have the smallest sample size?

a. A
b. B
c. C
d. D
e. E

49. Which study has a p value > 0.05?

a. A
b. B
c. C
d. D
e. E

50. Which study appears to be the most precise?

a. A
b. B
c. C
d. D
e. E

Items 51–53

Five new herpes simplex virus type 2–specific serologies are developed by different research laboratories. The test performance characteristics are used to create the receiver operator curve (ROC) illustrated in the following figure.

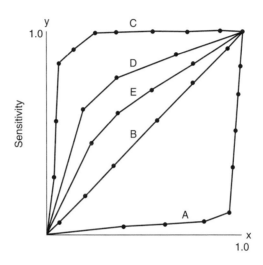

51. The x axis represents

a. True negatives
b. Prevalence of disease
c. False-negatives
d. False-positives
e. Positive predictive values

52. The main purpose of the ROC curves in the preceding example is to

a. Determine cut-off points for a new test
b. Compare the diagnostic accuracy of the new tests
c. Assess the utility of a new test in a low-prevalence population
d. Determine the test performance characteristics
e. Determine the cost-effectiveness of a new test

53. Which of the five tests would be best to use as a diagnostic tool?

a. A
b. B
c. C
d. D
e. E

54. A decision analysis is undertaken in an attempt to determine which approach, radiation therapy or surgery, is best for the management of prostate cancer. A sensitivity analysis is plotted on the graph shown in the following figure. The x axis represents the probability of death from surgery, and the y axis represents the life expectancy ("expected utility") expressed in quality-adjusted life years (QALYs).

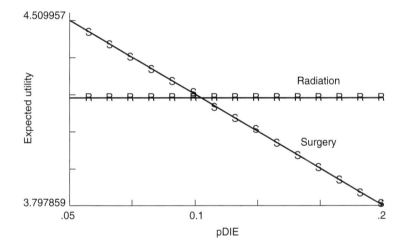

Based on this information, you conclude that

a. Radiation therapy is always the best approach
b. Surgery is always the best approach
c. Radiation therapy is the best approach when mortality from surgery exceeds 11%
d. Mortality from surgery does not affect the choice of approach
e. Surgery is the preferred approach when mortality from the procedure exceeds 20%

55. A prospective cohort study examining the association between passive smoking and cervical cancer reveals an odd ratio of 1.3 (95% confidence interval 0.8–5.6). The most appropriate conclusion is that

a. There is a significant association between passive smoking and cervical cancer
b. The null hypothesis is rejected
c. There is a type 1 error
d. The α was set at 0.10
e. A 90% confidence interval would result in a narrower confidence interval

56. Consider the following two-way scatter plot examining the relationship between glomerular filtration rate (GFR) on the y axis and the reciprocal of plasma creatinine (1/Cr) on the x axis.

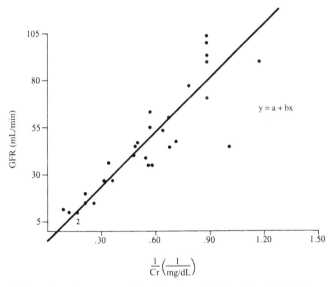

(Adapted, with permission, from Ingelfinger JA, Mosteller F, Thibodeau LA, Ware JH. *Biostatistics in Clinical Medicine,* 3rd ed. New York, McGraw-Hill, 1994: 205.)

This is an example of

a. A correlation analysis with a coefficient between 0 and 1
b. A logistic regression analysis
c. A simple linear regression analysis
d. A multiple regression analysis
e. A correlation analysis with a coefficient between −1 and 0

57. Consider the results of two hypothetical intervention studies:

	Study A	Study B
Incidence of mortality in the control group	1.3%	20%
Incidence of mortality in the intervention group	0.6%	9.2%

What is the most useful measure of association in assessing the clinical relevance of these two studies?

a. The relative risk (RR)
b. The relative risk reduction (RRR)
c. The odd ratio (OR)
d. The attributable risk reduction (ARR)
e. The numbers needed to treat (NNT)

58. A hypothetical study examining the association between serum cholesterol (>280) and cardiovascular disease (CVD) demonstrates a crude relative risk of 3.0. When the data is stratified by gender, the relative risk for men is 4.0 and the relative risk for women is 1.0. The adjusted risk is 3.0. The most appropriate interpretation of the results of this study is that

a. Gender is both a confounder and an effect modifier
b. Gender is a confounder only
c. Gender is an effect modifier only
d. Gender is neither a confounder nor an effect modifier
e. Gender is a causal pathway

59. A clinical training program wishes to evaluate the reliability of self-assessment of clinical skills as a tool for measuring improvement. After a teaching session, students are asked to rank themselves (on a scale of 1 to 5) on 10 examination procedures. The preceptor also ranks the students according to the same scale. The results of the two assessments are then compared. The most appropriate test statistic to compare results is

a. A Kappa statistics test
b. A student t test
c. A Wilcoxon rank sum test
d. A chi-square test
e. A correlation analysis

60. Which of the following tests can be used to study ordinal data from two independent samples from a population that is not normally distributed?

a. The student t test
b. The Wilcoxon rank sum test
c. The chi-square test
d. The one-way analysis of variance
e. The Mantel-Haenszel method

61. Point prevalence studies tend to overestimate the occurrence of which of the following diseases?

a. Diseases with a high incidence
b. Diseases with a long duration
c. Diseases with a high mortality
d. Diseases with a short duration
e. Diseases with a low incidence

62. Consider the following study assessing the proportion of patients presenting with urethritis who were tested for *Chlamydia trachomatis* (CT) at two different health centers:

Health Center	CT Test Yes	No
A	220	100
B	150	80

The data is analyzed using the chi-square distribution to determine if there is a significant difference in proportions between the two health centers. How many degrees of freedom should be used for this distribution?

a. 1
b. 2
c. 3
d. 4
e. 6

63. Consider the following survival curve for women diagnosed with disease XYZ.

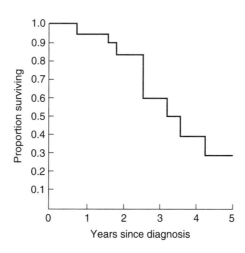

This curve suggests that the five-year survival rate is

a. 10%
b. 20%
c. 30%
d. 40%
e. 50%

Items 64–67

For each of the following descriptions, match the appropriate measure of frequency.

a. Fetal mortality
b. Infant mortality
c. Perinatal mortality
d. Neonatal mortality
e. Postneonatal mortality
f. Maternal mortality

64. Number of deaths in the first 28 days of life per 1000 live births in 1 year. (**SELECT 1 RATE**)

65. Number of fetal deaths plus deaths in the first week of life per 1000 total births in 1 year. (**SELECT 1 RATE**)

66. Number of deaths under the age of 1 year per 1000 live births in 1 year. (**SELECT 1 RATE**)

67. Number of deaths between the ages of 28 days and 11 months per 1000 live births in 1 year. (**SELECT 1 RATE**)

Items 68–69

For each of the following questions, choose the appropriate epidemiologic term it refers to.

a. Internal validity
b. External validity
c. Precision
d. Power
e. Statistical significance

68. A study demonstrates that the risk of cardiovascular disease among physicians can be reduced by aspirin intake. Can the results of this study be applied to the population at large?

69. An intervention study demonstrates that attending a sexual history–taking skills-building workshop increases the level of comfort of providers in questioning patients about the number of sexual partners (RR = 1.4, 95% CI 1.2–33.8). Are the results of the study reliable?

DIRECTIONS: Each group of questions below consists of lettered options followed by numbered items. For each numbered item, select the appropriate lettered option(s). Each lettered option may be used once, more than once, or not at all. Choose exactly the number of options indicated following each item.

Items 70–73

For each of the studies below, choose the most appropriate statistical test to analyze the data.

a. Chi-square analysis
b. Student t test
c. Paired t test
d. Analysis of variance
e. Linear regression
f. Multiple regression
g. Correlation analysis
h. McNemar test

70. Comparison of systolic blood pressures in independent samples of pregnant and nonpregnant women. **(SELECT 1 TEST)**

71. Comparison of the prevalence of hepatitis B surface antigen (HBsAg) in medical and dental students. **(SELECT 1 TEST)**

72. Comparison of the level of blood glucose in male and female rats following administration of three different drugs. **(SELECT 1 TEST)**

73. Comparison of serum cholesterol before and after ingestion of hamburgers in a sample of fast-food patrons. **(SELECT 1 TEST)**

Items 74–77

For each of the following descriptions, pick the appropriate epidemiologic term.

a. Confounding
b. Effect modification
c. Differential misclassification
d. Lead-time bias
e. Selection bias
f. Nondifferential misclassification

74. Elevated bilirubin levels in neonates are associated with brain damage only in babies who also have infections or severe hemolytic disease. **(SELECT 1 TERM)**

75. People who drink coffee tend to smoke more, and for this reason coffee drinkers have a higher risk of lung cancer. **(SELECT 1 TERM)**

76. Higher lead levels in hyperactive children may be due to increased consumption of paint in children who were already hyperactive. **(SELECT 1 TERM)**

77. A prospective cohort study with an imprecise measurement of exposure to radiation fails to demonstrate a significant association with cancer. **(SELECT 1 TERM)**

Items 78–81

In each statement below, data are presented based on a cohort study of coronary heart disease. Choose the parameter that best describes each of these statements.
a. Point prevalence
b. Cumulative incidence
c. Standardized morbidity ratio
d. Relative risk
e. Incidence density
f. Odds ratio
g. Case fatality rate

78. At the initial examination, 17 persons per 1000 had evidence of coronary heart disease (CHD). **(SELECT 1 PARAMETER)**

79. Among a cohort of heavy smokers, the observed frequency of angina pectoris was 1.6 times as great as the expected frequency during the first 12 years of the study. **(SELECT 1 PARAMETER)**

80. During the first eight years of the study, 45 persons developed coronary heart disease per 1000 persons who entered the study free of disease. **(SELECT 1 PARAMETER)**

81. At the end of the study, a total of 129 nonfatal myocardial infarctions per 54,560 person-years of observation occurred in the study population. **(SELECT 1 PARAMETER)**

Items 82–86

Match the examples below with the appropriate epidemiologic terms.
a. Lead-time bias
b. Surveillance bias
c. Recall bias
d. Type 1 error
e. Power
f. Length time bias
g. Confounding

82. Medical students who fail a physiology examination are more likely to report missing two or more physiology lectures than those who fail a neuroanatomy examination. **(SELECT 1 TERM)**

83. The chance of discovering the truth that twice as many of your friends are at the movies as are studying for their board examinations. **(SELECT 1 TERM)**

84. In a class of 150 medical students, there will likely be a few who can answer this question correctly without understanding the material. **(SELECT 1 TERM)**

85. The likelihood of finding a lost biochemistry notebook in your apartment is higher in the month of June than in the month of March. (SELECT 1 TERM)

86. Medical students enrolled in a first-year anatomy class are more likely to remain at their same addresses for the next two years than medical students enrolled in fourth-year clerkships. (SELECT 1 TERM)

Items 87–90

Choose the rate that best describes each statement below.
a. Secondary attack rate
b. Case fatality rate
c. Morbidity rate
d. Age-adjusted mortality
e. Crude mortality

87. Death occurs in 10% of cases of meningococcal meningitis. (SELECT 1 RATE)

88. Approximately 9 people die each year in the United States for every 1000 estimated to be alive. (SELECT 1 RATE)

89. Eighty percent of susceptible household contacts of a child with chicken pox develop this disease. (SELECT 1 RATE)

90. Children between the ages of 1 and 5 have an average of eight colds per year. (SELECT 1 RATE)

Items 91–94

Choose the term that best fits the description.
a. Matching
b. Stratification
c. Age adjustment
d. Multivariate statistical analysis
e. Survival analysis

91. In a cohort study of hypertensive men, the proportions of subjects with high and low renin levels who survived for five years are compared separately among those aged 40 to 49, those aged 50 to 59, and those aged 60 to 69 at entry. (SELECT 1 TERM)

92. A sampling strategy is used to achieve comparability of the groups being studied. (SELECT 1 TERM)

93. A technique that takes into account variable length of follow-up is used. (SELECT 1 TERM)

94. Six different risk ratios are calculated: one for each sex at each of three social class levels. (SELECT 1 TERM)

Items 95–98

For each of the studies described, select the reason for which the conclusion can be misleading or false.

a. Lack of a control group
b. Lack of proper follow-up
c. Lack of adjustment for age
d. Lack of denominators
e. Lack of adjustment for race

95. Of 250 consecutive, unselected women in whom acute cholecystitis was diagnosed, 75 were under age 50 and 175 were over age 50. The investigator concluded that older women are at greater risk of acute cholecystitis than are younger women. (**SELECT 1 ERROR**)

96. In a review of 3000 patients in whom adult-onset diabetes was diagnosed, 2000 of these patients were obese at the time of diagnosis. The investigator concluded that there is an association between diabetes and obesity. (**SELECT 1 ERROR**)

97. Acute anxiety neurosis was diagnosed among 250 patients and follow-up data were available on 80% of these patients 10 years later. The mortality experience of this cohort was no different from that of the general population. The authors concluded that the diagnosis of acute anxiety neurosis is not associated with a decrease in longevity. (**SELECT 1 ERROR**)

98. Of 143 patients who died of bacterial endocarditis and on whom autopsies were performed, 2% were less than 10 years of age. The authors concluded that bacterial endocarditis is rare in childhood. (**SELECT 1 ERROR**)

Items 99–102

Consider the following decision tree assessing radiation therapy versus surgery for the treatment of prostate cancer: The expected utility, life expectancy, is expressed in quality-adjusted life years, or QALYs.

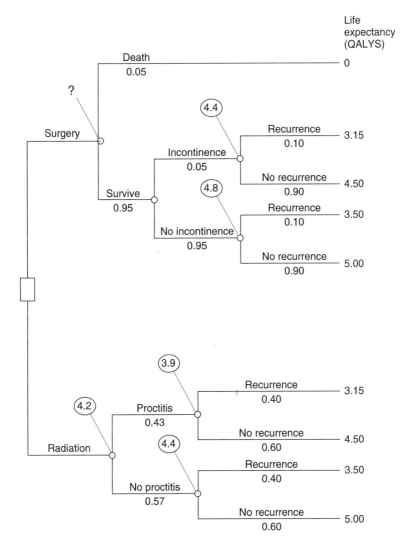

99. Which of the following statements is true concerning the creation of a decision tree used for clinical decision making?

a. The first nodes in a tree are chance nodes
b. Branches from the chance nodes must be mutually exclusive and collectively exhaustive
c. The terminal nodes represent prevalence of disease
d. The expected utilities are calculated by folding back the tree from left to right
e. The numerical values of the expected utility are expressed in different units than the expected outcomes

100. The quality-adjusted life expectancy for surgery is

a. $(4.4 + 4.8) \times 0.95 = 8.74$
b. $(4.4 \times 0.95) + (4.8 \times 0.05) = 4.42$
c. $[(4.4 \times 0.05) + (4.8 \times 0.95)] \times 0.95 = 4.5$
d. $(4.4 \times 0.95) + (4.8 \times 0.95) = 8.74$
e. $(4.4 \times 0.90) + (4.8 \times 0.90) = 8.28$

101. Based on the results of this decision analysis, which approach appears preferable?

a. Surgery
b. Radiation
c. Surgery, only if there is no probability of death
d. Radiation followed by surgery, if there is a recurrence
e. No preferable approach can be identified

102. If radiation therapy was *never* associated with the complication of proctitis, the quality-adjusted life expectancy would be

a. 5.0
b. 3.5
c. $(3.5 + 5.0)/2 = 4.25$
d. $(3.15 \times 0.4) + (4.5 \times 0.6) = 3.96$
e. $(3.5 \times 0.4) + (5.0 \times 0.6) = 4.4$

Items 103–106

The following 2×2 table represents the findings of a five-year cohort study in which the incidence of suicide in veterans who served in Vietnam was compared with that of veterans who served elsewhere. Match the name of the parameter below with the appropriate formula.

	Suicide	**No Suicide**
Served in Vietnam	a	b
Served elsewhere	c	d

a. ad/bc
b. $(a + b)/(a + b + c + d)$
c. $(a + c)/(a + b + c + d)$
d. $[a/(a + b)]/[c/(c + d)]$
e. $[a/(a + b)] - [c/(c + d)]$

103. The odds ratio. (**SELECT 1 FORMULA**)

104. The relative risk. (**SELECT 1 FORMULA**)

105. The excess risk of suicide in Vietnam veterans. **(SELECT 1 FORMULA)**

106. The overall incidence (per five years) of suicide in the study. **(SELECT 1 FORMULA)**

Items 107–110

Match each description of a sampling procedure with the correct term.
a. Systematic sampling
b. Paired sampling
c. Simple random sampling
d. Stratified sampling
e. Cluster sampling

107. Each individual of the total group has an equal chance of being selected. **(SELECT 1 PROCEDURE)**

108. Households are selected at random, and every person in each household is included in the sample. **(SELECT 1 PROCEDURE)**

109. Individuals are initially assembled according to some order in a group and then individuals are selected according to some constant determinant; for instance, every fourth subject is selected. **(SELECT 1 PROCEDURE)**

110. Individuals are divided into subgroups on the basis of specified characteristics and then random samples are selected from each subgroup. **(SELECT 1 PROCEDURE)**

Items 111–115

A new test for chlamydial infections of the cervix is introduced. Half of the women who are tested have a positive test. Compared with the gold standard of careful cultures, 45% of those with a positive test are infected with chlamydia, and 95% of those with a negative test are free of the infection. Match the epidemiologic terms below with the correct percentage.
a. 25%
b. 45%
c. 63%
d. 90%
e. 95%

111. Sensitivity of the test. **(SELECT 1 PERCENTAGE)**

112. Specificity of the test. **(SELECT 1 PERCENTAGE)**

113. Prevalence of chlamydial infection in that community. **(SELECT 1 PERCENTAGE)**

114. Predictive value of a positive test. **(SELECT 1 PERCENTAGE)**

115. Predictive value of a negative test. **(SELECT 1 PERCENTAGE)**

Items 116–119

For each result or conclusion described below, select the choice that might best explain it.

a. Ecologic fallacy
b. Type 1 error
c. Type 2 error
d. Selection bias
e. Misclassification bias

116. A randomized blinded trial of aspirin to prevent myocardial infarction fails to find a difference between aspirin and placebo groups after five years ($N = 500$ per group; $p = 0.11$). **(SELECT 1 ERROR)**

117. A study of patterns of contraceptive use finds that counties with the highest per capita use of condoms also have the highest pregnancy rates ($N = 100,000$; $p < 0.001$) and concludes that condoms are ineffective as contraceptives. **(SELECT 1 ERROR)**

118. An investigator analyzes data from the National Health Interview Survey and finds that there is a positive association between consumption of turkey and degenerative joint disease in black women 50 to 59 years old ($N = 50$; $p < 0.05$). **(SELECT 1 ERROR)**

119. In a case-control study of lung cancer, cases' spouses are chosen as controls. The odds ratio for smoking is 3.0, which does not quite reach statistical significance ($N = 30$ per group; $p = 0.07$). **(SELECT 1 ERROR)**

Items 120–124

For each variable described below, choose the type of measurement scale.

a. Dichotomous scale
b. Nominal scale
c. Ordinal scale
d. Interval scale
e. Ratio scale

120. Survival of a particular patient for at least five years. **(SELECT 1 SCALE)**

121. Frequency of somnolence during biochemistry lectures: never, sometimes, usually, or always. **(SELECT 1 SCALE)**

122. Birth weight. **(SELECT 1 SCALE)**

123. Type of medical specialty. **(SELECT 1 SCALE)**

124. Year of birth. **(SELECT 1 SCALE)**

Items 125–127

Dr. Vera Blues, a noted psychiatric epidemiologist, is interested in the diagnosis of depression. She develops a new test for its diagnosis, which she calls the Blues test. According to the gold standard, which involves meeting the *DSM-IV* criteria, about 10% of adults in the United States are depressed. Dr. Blues applies her new test to 100 persons diagnosed as being depressed by the gold standard; 80 have a positive Blues test. She finds 400 persons who are not depressed; 60 have a positive test. She reports her findings in the *Journal of the Society of Academic Psychiatrists* (JSAP). Match the statements that Dr. Blues made in her article with the appropriate percentage.

a. 85%
b. 80%
c. 60%
d. 6%
e. <10%

125. "The specificity of the Blues test was ____." (SELECT 1 PERCENTAGE)

126. "The likelihood that someone with depression would have a positive Blues test was ____." (SELECT 1 PERCENTAGE)

127. "The likelihood that someone in the population with a negative Blues test would be depressed was ____." (SELECT 1 PERCENTAGE)

Items 128–130

Consider the following portion of a decision tree assessing the screening strategies with different tests for *Chlamydia trachomatis.*

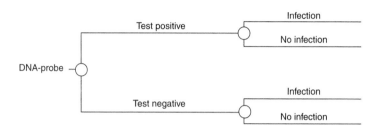

For each probability described below, select the most appropriate definition.

a. True positives
b. Prevalence of disease
c. True positives + false-positives
d. True positives + false-negatives
e. True negatives + false-negatives
f. True negatives + false-positives
g. Positive predictive value
h. Negative predictive value
i. 1– negative predictive value
j. 1– positive predictive value

128. The probability of a positive DNA-probe. (**SELECT 1 DEFINITION**)

129. The probability of infection if the DNA-probe is negative. (**SELECT 1 DEFINITION**)

130. The probability of no infection if the DNA-probe is positive. (**SELECT 1 DEFINITION**)

BIOSTATISTICS AND METHODS OF EPIDEMIOLOGY

Answers

1. The answer is d. *(Rosner, 5/e, pp 46–52. Greenberg, 2/e, pp 76–79.)* The multiplicative rule applies to independent events. The probability of a negative test if there is cancer can be expressed as p (test$^-$ / disease$^+$) and is equal to $1-$ sensitivity $(1 - 0.9 = 0.1)$, or the false-negative rate. The probability of two negative consecutive tests is $(0.1)(0.1) = 0.01 = 1/100$. The probability that a woman who has cancer will test negative decreases with the number of mammographies done. This is inherent to the sensitivity of the test. The higher the sensitivity, the lower the probability of false-negative tests as they are repeated.

2. The answer is c. *(Greenberg, 2/e, pp 106–109.)* This study is a prospective cohort study because the subjects (pregnant women) were categorized on the basis of exposure or lack of exposure to a risk factor (smoking during pregnancy), and then were followed to determine if a particular outcome (low-birth-weight babies) resulted. The term *cohort* refers to the group of subjects who are followed forward in time to see which ones develop the outcome. Clinical trials are prospective studies in which an intervention is applied—no intervention was mentioned in the question: it would be unethical to assign one or the other group to smoking. In a case-control study of the relationship between low birth weight and maternal smoking, infants would be selected on the basis of low birth weight (cases) and normal birth weight (controls) and then the frequency of maternal smoking would be compared in the two groups. In cross-sectional studies, exposure and outcome are measured at the same point in time. A retrospective cohort study is similar in design to a prospective cohort study (subjects are chosen on the basis of exposure then assessed for outcome): the difference is that both the exposure and outcome have occurred when the study is undertaken. An example would be if you reviewed charts in a clinic the previous year, classified women as smokers or nonsmokers based on record documentation, and then looked at the birth weight of the children in both groups.

3. The answer is b. *(Ingelfinger, 3/e, pp 198–202.)* Although hypertension can resolve spontaneously, this is an unlikely explanation for resolution over a two-week period in 35% of the subjects. A much more likely explanation is regression toward the mean. Because of random fluctuations, any one measurement of blood pressure may be far from a person's normal blood pressure. By referring patients for the study based on a *single* measurement, those in whom the measurement was high (which proved later not to reflect the actual BP) are much more likely to be referred than those in whom the measurement was too low. Thus, in any group selected based on a characteristic with substantial day-to-day variation, many will have values closer to the population mean when the measurement is repeated and the "worst patients" will improve. Neither baseline drift (which occurs with measurements on certain machines that require frequent calibration) nor measurement error is as likely an explanation. The Hawthorne effect refers to a tendency among study subjects to change simply because they are being studied. It is much more likely to affect studies of behavior or attitudes than a study of blood pressure.

4. The answer is d. *(Greenberg, 2/e, pp 18–19.)* Person-years of observation are frequently used in the denominator of incidence rates and provide a method of dealing with variable follow-up periods. Person-years of observation simultaneously take into account the number of persons under observation and the duration of observation of each person. For example, if eight new cases of diabetes occurred among 1000 people followed for two years, the incidence would be 8 cases per 2000 person-years, or 4 per 1000 person-years of follow-up. The distinction between rates and proportions is not well maintained in standard epidemiologic terminology. Rates should have units of inverse time and will vary depending on the units of measurement of time; they can vary from 0 to infinity. However, such terms as *case fatality rate, attack rate,* and *prevalence rate* are in widespread usage even though technically they are all proportions; that is, they vary between 0 and 1 and are unitless.

5. The answer is d. *(Rosner, 5/e, p 125.)* For any normal distribution, 68% of the population values are contained within the interval of the mean $\pm$ 1 standard deviation (16% will be higher and 16% will be lower), 95% within the mean ± 2 standard deviations (2.5% will be higher and 2.5% will be lower), and 99% within the mean ± 3 standard deviations (0.5% will be higher and 0.5% will be lower). In this case, 59.5 kg is equal to the mean ± 1 standard deviation, which means 16% of women will be heavier.

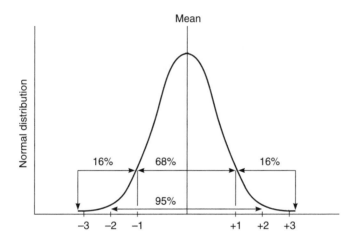

6. The answer is e. *(Rosner, 5/e, pp 9–16.)* The correct values for mean, median, and mode are 3.4, 3, and 2. The mean is the average: the sum of the observations divided by the number of observations. In this case, the mean is 31/9 = 3.4. The median is the middle observation in a series of ordered observations, that is, the 50th percentile. In this case, there is an uneven number (9) of observations. When the observations are ordered— 1, 2, 2, 2, 3, 4, 4, 6, 7—the median is 3. If the number of observations is even, it is midway between the two middle observations. For example, if we were to have only 8 observations such as : 1, 2, 2, 2, 3, 4, 6, 7, then the median would be equal to the average of the fourth and fifth largest observations: 2 + 3/2 = 2.5. The mode is the observation that occurs with greatest frequency; in this case it is 2, which occurs three times.

7. The answer is c. *(Rosner, 5/e, pp 371–373.)* The chi-square is used for categorical data if no cell has an expected count less than 1, and no more than 20% of the cells have an expected count less than 5. In this case, the expected counts are 4.2 ($10 \times 8/19$) for cell a, 5.7 ($10 \times 11/19$) for cell b, 3.7 ($9 \times 8/19$) for cell c, and 5.2 ($9 \times 11/19$) for cell d. Because 50% of the cells have an expected count of less than 5, the Fisher's exact test is appropriate. In general, it is used when the sample size is small. The McNemar's test is used for paired dichotomous (one of two distinct values such as male or female; no fraction is possible) data, the student *t* test for independent continuous (where fractions are possible such as weight [55.2 kg], cholesterol levels, etc.) data, and the analysis of variance for analysis of several independent means.

8. The answer is d. (*Greenberg, 2/e, p 18.*) According to the table, 10 new cases of tuberculosis developed among the 500 persons belonging to households with a case of tuberculosis at the time of the first survey. Because these 500 persons were followed for 2 years, the number of person-years of exposure is 1000. Therefore, the incidence rate is calculated as follows:

$$\frac{10 \text{ new cases}}{500 \text{ persons} \times 2 \text{ years}} = 10 \text{ cases per 1000 person-years}$$

9. The answer is c. (*Greenberg, 2/e, p 18.*) Ten new cases of tuberculosis developed among 10,000 persons belonging to households that had no culture-positive cases at the time of the first survey. Since these 10,000 persons were followed for 2 years, the number of person-years of exposure is 20,000. Therefore, the incidence rate is calculated as follows:

$$\frac{10 \text{ new cases}}{10,000 \text{ persons} \times 2 \text{ years}} = 0.5 \text{ cases per 1000 person-years}$$

10. The answer is e. (*Greenberg, 2/e, pp 98–99.*) The relative risk is the ratio of the incidence of a disease in a group exposed to a factor (in this case, household contact with tuberculosis) to the incidence in a group not exposed to the factor (persons without household contact). Therefore, the relative risk is

$$\frac{\text{Incidence in households with exposure}}{\text{Incidence in households without exposure}} = \frac{10}{0.5} = 20$$

Identification of groups with a high level of relative risk can be useful in planning disease control programs.

11. The answer is e. *(Greenberg, 2/e, p 106.)* In experimental studies, the investigators determine exposure of the study and control groups to a suspected causal factor and measure responses in the two groups. In observational studies, investigators have no control over exposure to a suspected causal factor but can measure responses in those who are and are not exposed. In both types of studies, the attempt is made to use study and control groups similar in regard to all variables except exposure to the factor under study.

12. The answer is c. *(Greenberg, 2/e, pp 136–140, 123–126.)* Recall bias, a form of information bias and differential misclassification, occurs when cases are more likely to recall past events than controls. Indeed, persons experiencing a bad outcome may be more likely to search their past (and prod their memory) about potential causes for the occurrence. This is a particular problem with case-control studies. Recall bias could cause a falsely high odds ratio; it is potentially a problem when using maternal recall to investigate exposures associated with birth defects. In this case, mothers with children with undescended testes may be more accurate in quantifying smoking habits. Because this misclassification of exposure is not random in both the case and controls, it is termed differential misclassification. Nondifferential misclassification occurs when the memory of an exposure is unrelated to the fact that a person has a disease or not. It is often the consequence of an imprecise measurement of exposure (remembering specific nutrition information that occurred many months ago). The important point to remember is that differential misclassification may result in an overestimate of an association while nondifferential misclassification nearly always causes the results to move toward the null (no association). Selection bias refers to systematic errors in the way subjects are included in a study. Confounding occurs when the apparent effect of an exposure is partly or entirely due to a third factor associated with both exposure and outcome. Although a third factor could potentially be present, it has not been identified here, and the major concern in this case should be the recall bias.

13. The answer is b. *(Rosner, 5/e, pp 181–183, 219.)* Since undescended testes are uncommon, the odds ratio in this study approximates the relative risk (risk ratio). The fact that the 95% confidence interval excludes 1.0

means that p is less than 0.05. Confidence intervals describe the range of values not significantly different from the observed value, with a type 1 error rate (alpha) of 1.0 minus the level of confidence. Thus, a 95% confidence interval shows the numbers that are not significantly different statistically from what was observed at the 5% level. The lower the level of confidence, the narrower the confidence interval, so a 90% confidence interval would be narrower than a 95% confidence interval, in this case excluding 1.0 for certain. Thus, if the study is accurate, it suggests that baby boys whose mothers smoke are 2.6 times as likely to have undescended testes. A larger sample size decreases variability, thus decreasing the confidence interval.

14. The answer is d. (*Rosner, 5/e, pp 52–55.*) For two events or conditions, the probability that either will occur is the sum of their probabilities, minus the probability that both will occur. This is illustrated in the following figure.

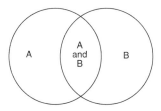

If we simply add the probability of A to the probability of B, the area labeled "A and B" will get counted twice. Therefore, the probability of (A and B) must be subtracted from the sum of the probabilities: p (A or B) = p (A) + p (B) − p (A and B). In this question, it is specifically stated that the two conditions are independent. When that is the case, the probability that both will occur is the product of their probabilities: p (A and B) = p A × p B. The answer to this problem is 0.1 + 0.5 − (0.1)(0.5) = 0.55. Note that another common situation is when two conditions are mutually exclusive rather than independent (i.e., the probability that both will occur is zero). In this case, the probability that either one will occur is simply the sum of their probabilities. For example, if condition A were blue eyes and condition B brown eyes, the probability of either blue or brown eyes would be 0.60.

15. The answer is e. (*Greenberg, 2/e, pp 119–121.*) Case-control studies are well suited to studying rare disorders with multiple potential causes. They are also quickly mounted and conducted and are less expensive than prospective studies. The large database will enhance selection of a control group. A retrospective cohort study requires that you identify the exposed and the unexposed from years back and that you follow them over time. It is unsuited for rare cancers, and not applicable to the data you have available.

16. The answer is b. *(Greenberg, 2/e, pp 80–81. USPS Task Force, 2/e, p xlv.)* Rapidly progressive cancers will be less likely to be detected by a screening test if symptoms rapidly develop because the window period between the time the cancer can be detected when it is asymptomatic by a screening test and the time it will become clinically apparent is short. This is described as *length bias.* Screening tests are more effective in terms of prolonging life (or other desirable outcomes) when they are used to detect more slowly growing tumors. Lead-time bias occurs when the screening test advances the time of diagnosis, but no true prolongation of life occurs because survival for persons who are screened and those who are not is the same from the time the cancer occurs. Information bias occurs when there is a systematic difference in the way data are collected (inaccurate or imprecise measure) for either the exposure or the outcome. Recall bias is one form of information bias (see answer for question 12) and refers to what one may remember for an exposure, so it is irrelevant here. Selection bias occurs when the inclusion of a subject in a study group is linked to the exposure of interest. As an example for a case-control study, if women who use oral contraceptives are suspected more often of having deep vein thrombosis (DVT), they would be hospitalized more often for evaluation and diagnosed more often than controls. Selection bias can also occur in cohort studies and is related to differential loss to follow-up. Surveillance bias refers to overdetection of the disease of interest because one of the groups goes to the doctor (or has a diagnostic test) more often than does another group. For example, women who take postmenopausal estrogens presumably go to the doctor (and probably have mammograms) more frequently than women who do not; thus, women who take estrogens may be more likely to have breast cancers detected because of the increased surveillance.

17. The answer is b. *(Greenberg, 2/e, pp 76–79.)* Sensitivity and specificity are measures of how often a diagnostic test gives the correct answer. Sensitivity reflects the test's performance in people who have the disease, and specificity measures the test's performance in people who do not have the disease. These definitions can be illustrated as follows:

	Disease Present	Disease Absent
Test positive	True positive (TP)	False-positive (FP)
Test negative	False-negative (FN)	True negative (TN)
Sensitivity = TP / (TP + FN)	Specificity = TN/(TN + FP)	

Among people who have the disease, there are two possibilities: either the test correctly identifies them (TP), or it falsely classifies them as negative (FN). Thus, among those with disease, sensitivity measures how often the test gives the right answer. (A good way to remember sensitivity is by the initials PID: positive in disease.) Similarly, among people who do not have the disease, there are also two possibilities: either the test will correctly identify them as not having disease (TN), or it will falsely classify them as diseased (FP). Thus, specificity measures how often the test gives the right answer among those who do not have the disease. (A good way to remember specificity is by the initials NIH: negative in health.)

As opposed to sensitivity and specificity, which measure the test's performance in groups of patients who do and do not have the disease, predictive value measures how often the test is right in patients grouped another way: by whether the test result is positive or negative. Thus, predictive value of a positive test is the proportion of positive tests that are true positives [TP/(TP + FP)], and predictive value of a negative result is the proportion of negative test results that are true negatives [TN/(TN + FN)].

But predictive value is a little tricky because it also depends on the prevalence of the disease in the population tested. In this case, Dr. Stewells assembled groups of 100 patients with and without cholera, and the prevalence is not given. Therefore, predictive value cannot be calculated in this question, and the correct answer is B, since specificity is 88%, not 12%.

18. The answer is c. (*Greenberg, 2/e, pp 76–78. Rosner, 5/e, pp 58–60.*) In this study of 1000 patients with profuse diarrhea, 343 of them had cholera. Thus, the prevalence of cholera (in this population) was 343/1000. (Note that this is not an incidence because we are measuring cases at a specific point in time, rather than new cases that occur over a period of time.) The predictive value of a positive result can thus be directly determined as TP/(TP + FP) = 312/(312 + 79) = 80%. Similarly, the predictive value of a negative result is TN/(TN + FN) = 578/(578 + 31) = 95%. Note here that this predictive value refers to the predictive value of the test in patients admitted to the hospital with profuse diarrhea. Since prevalence data from the general population are still lacking, the usefulness of this test in the general population is undefined. Predictably, the positive predictive value of this test in an asymptomatic population will be less.

19. The answer is b. *(Greenberg, 2/e, p 83.)* As the prevalence falls, more and more of those tested will not have cholera. This would change neither the sensitivity nor specificity of the test, which do not depend on disease prevalence, but would affect predictive value: as prevalence falls, predictive value of a positive result also falls, whereas predictive value of a negative result rises. This makes sense: as a disease becomes more and more unlikely, positive test results should be viewed with increasing skepticism, whereas negative results become increasingly believable.

20. The answer is a. *(Greenberg, 2/e, pp 91–93.)* Randomization is the use of a predetermined plan of allocation or assignment of subjects to treatment groups such that assignment occurs solely by chance. It is used to eliminate bias on the part of the investigator and the subject in the choice of treatment group. The goal of randomization is to allow chance to distribute unknown sources of biologic variability equally to the treatment and control groups. However, because chance does determine assignment, significant differences between the groups may arise, especially if the number of subjects is small. Therefore, whenever randomization is used, the comparability of the treatment groups should be assessed to determine whether or not balance was achieved

21. The answer is d. *(Greenberg, 2/e, pp 121–126.)* The study described was a case-control study. In this type of study, people who have a disease (cases) are compared with people whom they closely resemble except for the presence of the disease under study (controls). Cases and controls are then studied for the frequency of exposure to a suspected risk factor. In case-control studies, the validity of inferences about the causal relationship between the exposure (cigarette smoking) and the disease (lung cancer) depends on how comparable the cases and controls are for all variables that may be related to both the risk factor and disease under study (e.g., age, sex, race, place of residence, and occupation). Matching is a method to control for confounding in case-control studies to eliminate the effect of any extraneous variable that is not under study but may have an effect on the results. In clinical trials, or experimental/intervention studies, the investigators allocate the exposure. Correlation studies are used to compare disease frequencies between entire populations (as opposed to individuals). For example, a correlation study could examine the consumption of animal fat and the rates of colon cancer among 20 different countries.

22–24. The answers are 22-b, 23-d, 24-a. *(Greenberg, 2/e, pp 113–115.)* The relative risk is defined as the incidence rate among the exposed (I_e) divided by the incidence rate among the nonexposed (I_o). In this case, $(120/100,000)/(10/100,000) = 12$. The attributable risk (AR) is defined as $I_e - I_o = (120/100,000) - (10/100,000) = 110/100,000$. The attributable risk percentage is equal to $[(I_e - I_o) / I_e] \times 100 = (110/100,000)/(120/100,000) = 92\%$. If the prevalence of smoking was reduced to 10%, 11/100,000 excess cases of lung cancer due to smoking could be averted. We can calculate this by using the population attributable risk (PAR), which is defined by the attributable risk x prevalence of exposure in the population. If the prevalence of smoking in the population is 20%, then the PAR is calculated as follows: AR $\times$ prevalence of exposure $= 110/100,00 \times 20/100 = 22/100,000$. If the prevalence of smoking is 10%, then AR $\times$ prevalence of exposure $= 110/100,000 \times 10/100 = 11/100,000$.

25. The answer is c. *(Greenberg, 2/e, pp 94–97. Hennekens, pp 206–208.)* Intent-to-treat analysis, that is including in the final results *all* the subjects who were initially randomized to receive either the drug or the placebo, is the preferred method of analysis for intervention studies. Although it may be tempting to include only those who complied with the medication, the results can be misleading. This study is a classic example of this pittfall. Indeed, the study showed that the difference in mortality between those who did and did not adhere to *placebo* was even greater: 15 versus 28%. The difference persisted even after controlling for 40 different confounders. Thus, something related to compliance (with either the medication or the placebo) appeared to decrease mortality. Therefore, as a rule, remember that once randomization has been performed, all participants, regardless of their compliance, should be included in the results.

26. The answer is b. (*Greenberg, 2/e, p 125.*) Matching is a technique used in the design of the study to control for confounding. Subjects enrolled in a study are matched for age, gender, smoking, or any variable that is not being analyzed. This technique is not used for large cohort studies as it would often be too time-consuming, restrictive, and expensive to find a match for each subject entering the study. Therefore, controlling for confounding is done in the analysis when a large group is recruited. Matching is mainly used when dealing with small case-control studies where the number of subjects enrolled would be too small to yield statistical results if stratified by subgroups. Randomization is used in clinical trials to control confounding (sample size needs to be large—see the answer to question 20). Matching cannot be used in correlation studies or cross-sectional studies: these are descriptive studies to assess disease occurrence and they do not have control groups to test a hypothesis.

27–28. The answers are 27-b, 28-a. (*Greenberg, 2/e, pp 94–97.*) In order to maximize compliance, a researcher can assess the compliance of subjects by giving them either the active or inert medication for a certain period of time, before the randomization for the study has occurred. Noncompliant persons can be dropped from the entire study population and the compliant persons are then randominzed to receive either active or inert medication (placebo). This technique was used for the physicians' health study to determine if the use of aspirin would reduce cardiovascular mortality. Keeping logs and frequent contacts from research staff can also help maintain compliance. The use of the placebo is to assess for responses that may simply be attributed to receiving an intervention, whether active or inert. It has been shown that even patients who receive inert medication can do better than if receiving nothing. Therefore, they need to represent the control group of any clinical trial to account for the "placebo effect." In a double-blinded study, both the investigators and the subjects are not aware of who is receiving active or inactive medication. This reduces the bias in the ascertainment of outcome. Intent-to-treat analysis refers to including *all* subjects who were initially randomized in the final analysis of results, compliers and noncompliers alike (see the answer to question 25). α and β error are used for statistical significance and do not affect the internal validity (i.e., are not a source of bias) of a study. Loss to follow-up, particularly if it is large or unequal between the intervention and control groups, can be a major source of bias for any prospective study, including clinical trials, if it is linked to the exposure, to the outcome, or both. As this study is likely to require a long follow-up period, every effort must be made to ensure complete follow-up. The incidence of lung cancer will not affect the internal validity of the study, but if it is low, it may affect the power of the study to measure differences between groups (because there may be an insufficient number of outcomes to reach statistical significance between the two groups).

29. The answer is e. *(Greenberg, 2/e, pp 49–53.)* Comparison of crude death rates of countries with different population compositions is fruitless. Adjusting both crude death rates to a standard population gives age-adjusted rates, which can be compared. Developed nations have higher crude death rates because larger proportions of their populations are elderly and thus have a higher probability of dying. Since rates account for population size, a larger population can be compared with a smaller one. Death rates are just one factor in evaluating health care systems.

30. The answer is b. *(Hennekens, pp 20–25.)* Because the association between the risk factor (use of smokeless tobacco) and the disease (oral lesions) is measured at a single point in time in a whole group of subjects, this is a cross-sectional study. A case-control study might be performed over a similar time period, but the sampling would be different: one sample would be selected from among those baseball players found to have oral lesions (the cases) and a separate sample would be selected from among those players whose mouths were normal (the controls). In a cohort study, the habits of a group of players initially free of the disease would be measured, and these players would be followed over time to see how many develop the lesions. A clinical trial involves allocation of the subjects by the investigator (usually randomly) to one of two or more treatment groups.

31. The answer is d. *(Greenberg, 2/e, p 18.)* Cross-sectional studies allow one to estimate the prevalence (the number of existing cases at one point in time divided by the population at risk) but not incidence (number of new cases occurring over a period of time divided by the population at risk and the period of time at risk). The prevalence of mouth lesions is 80/110 (73%) in the users of smokeless tobacco. The relative risk, the incidence density, and cumulative incidence rates all apply only to cohort studies where the occurrence of disease in initially healthy subjects is examined over time among the exposed and the nonexposed. The odds ratio applies to case-control studies and cross-sectional studies.

32. The answer is c. (*Hennekens, p 357.*) The chi-square test can be used for statistical analysis of categorical data (no fractions are possible; number of persons are categorized as ill or not ill, dead or alive, etc.; and data are often presented in 2 × 2 tables). The odds ratio can be used as a measure of association. In this case, it is equal to (80 × 34)/(30 × 2). Because the association between the risk factor (use of smokeless tobacco) and the disease (oral lesions) is measured at a single point in time in a whole group of subjects, no temporal association between the exposure and the outcome can be assessed. Furthermore, as this is not a cohort study in which subjects are chosen on the basis of exposure, there should be no expectations that the number of exposed persons would be similar to those who are not exposed.

33. The answer is c. (*Hennekens, pp 200–201.*) The importance of blinding, while it usually cannot be overemphasized, is not relevant in a study with total mortality as the end point: it is not possible to misclassify someone as alive when that person is really dead (except with fraudulent results). Power is not relevant in a study that shows a significant effect. If the results had failed to show a significant difference ($p > 0.05$) between the two groups, one may wonder whether the study had sufficient power. In a randomized study, the percentages of patients who actually had myocardial infarctions should be similar in the two groups. Total mortality is a much more important end point than mortality from coronary heart disease, but long-term follow-up is absolutely essential in determining whether a therapy is useful. Perhaps the new agent simply postpones mortality by a few days or weeks.

34. The answer is b. (*Greenberg, 2/e, pp 64–68.*) The secondary attack rate of a disease is the ratio of the number of cases of a specified disease among persons exposed to index cases divided by the total number so exposed. According to the data, 400 cases of pertussis occurred among 4000 fully immunized children who were exposed to a sibling who had the disease. The secondary attack rate, as a percentage, among fully immunized children after household exposure is, therefore,

$$\frac{400}{4000} \times 100\% = 10\%$$

35. The answer is c. *(Jekel, 1996, p 208.)* The efficacy of vaccine, or the percentage reduction in the incidence of disease in vaccinated compared with unvaccinated subjects, is given by the expression Protection = (incidence in unvaccinated − incidence in vaccinated)/incidence in unvaccinated = 100

$$\left[\left(\frac{400}{1000} \right) - \left(\frac{400}{4000} \right) \right] \Big/ \frac{400}{100} \times 100\% = 75\%$$

36. The answer is e. *(Greenberg, 2/e, pp 98–99.)* The relative risk is the ratio of the incidence rates of two groups who differ by some factor—in this instance, immunization status:

$$\frac{\text{Incidence rate among unimmunized children}}{\text{Incidence rate among fully immunized children}}$$

or

$$\frac{400 \text{ cases/1000 exposed children}}{400 \text{ cases/4000 exposed children}} = \frac{0.4}{0.1} = 4$$

37. The answer is d. *(Ingelfinger, 3/e, p 58.)* In decision analysis, *utilities* refer to the relative values placed on various outcomes that could be experienced by the *patients,* not the physicians. For example, perfect health might be assigned a utility of 100, and death assigned one of 0. What, then, would the utility be for life with moderate back pain? With careful questioning, one finds that most patients place a higher value on life with disability than would be anticipated. Different techniques can be used to have persons quantify utilities for a given outcome.

38. The answer is d. *(Hennekens, 2/e, pp 295–319.)* All the choices listed are methods to control for confounding. Matching and restriction (excluding smokers among cases and controls) can be achieved in the initial phase of designing the case-control study and *before* collecting information. Randomization is used for experimental studies. Once the data is collected, control for confounding can be performed in the analysis by stratification or multivariate analysis if there is a need to control for mutiple variables. In this example, we would first calculate the crude odds ratio from the 2 × 2 table including all cases and controls. We would then stratify the data by smoking status and calculate the odds ratio (OR) for each stratum (smokers and nonsmokers) as demonstrated in the following:

	All Subjects		Smokers		Nonsmokers	
	Dis +	Dis −	Dis +	Dis −	Dis +	Dis −
Drinker	a	b	a	b	a	b
Nondrinker	c	d	c	d	c	d
Crude (unadjusted) OR			ORs adjusted for smoking			

If the OR for the smokers and the nonsmokers is different than the *crude* OR, then confounding is present. In this situation, the *adjusted* OR would also be different than the crude OR.

39–41. The answers are 39-d, 40-c, 41-e. *(Greenberg, 2/e, p 18.)* The incidence of illness (as a percentage) is the total number of persons who have symptomatic illness divided by the total population at risk, and the calculation is (312 / 614) × 100% = 50.8%. The percentage of cases of German measles that were asymptomatic, or subclinical, is calculated by dividing the number of asymptomatic persons by the total number of infected persons. The calculation is [207 / (207 + 312)] × 100% = 39.9%. The information was stratified by age to determine if rates were similar. Age-specific infection rates were 90% in all age groups 0 to 59 years of age, while the rate was 10% in persons 60 years of age and over. The low attack rate in persons 60 and over suggests that this age group had developed immunity to German measles as a result of prior exposure at least 60 years before since there was uniform susceptibility in persons under 60.

42–44. The answers are 42-a, 43-d, 44-d. *(Greenberg, 2/e, pp 78–79. Hennekens, pp 331–335.)* There is a trade-off between sensitivity and specificity of a test because there is overlapping of the normal population and the population with disease for most screening tests. The interval 0 μg/dL to 30 μg/dL includes all values of the normal population, but also some values of the population with cancer; therefore, no value above 30 μg/dL will occur in individuals without disease. At this cut-off, the test will be 100% specific. However, you will miss some individuals with cancer, as some will have values between 20 μg/dL and 30 μg/dL. If the interval of 0 μg/dL to 25 μg/dL is chosen, then some persons with levels above 25 μg will have cancer and others will not. There will be some persons without cancer who will test positive (false-positives) and some persons with cancer will test negative (false-negatives). The last interval will be 100% sensitive as it will detect all cancers: there will be no false-negative tests. The trade-off is that it will be less specific: some persons without cancer will test positive (false-positive). Therefore, some confirmation of the test by another more specific method will be necessary before we can draw any conclusion.

45. The answer is e. *(Pagano, pp 15–24. Rosner, 5/e, pp 28–39.)* Line graphs are useful for presenting continuous data over time within different populations. In fact, in most cases, the horizontal axis scale in line graphs represents time in year, months, and so forth. Frequency polygons are used to illustrate frequency distributions for discrete or continuous data. More than one set of data can be superimposed for comparison. The horizontal axis often represents measure of the variable of interest (e.g., cholesterol) and the vertical axis represents the distribution either in numbers, relative frequency, or cumulative frequency. Histograms can also be used for this purpose, one set of data at a time. The horizontal axis should represent the true limits of intervals between data points (upper and lower limit) and the vertical axis should begin at zero. A bar chart is used to depict the frequency distribution of nominal or ordinal data. Only one set of data is represented for each chart. Pie charts can be used to illustrate relative frequencies of categorical data. (Note: all graphs represent hypothetical data.)

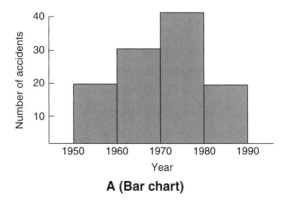

A (Bar chart)

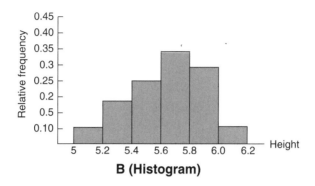

B (Histogram)

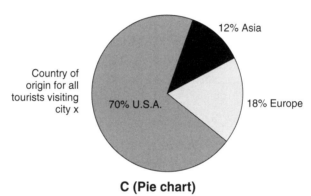

Country of origin for all tourists visiting city x

70% U.S.A.

12% Asia

18% Europe

C (Pie chart)

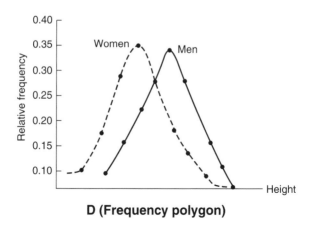

D (Frequency polygon)

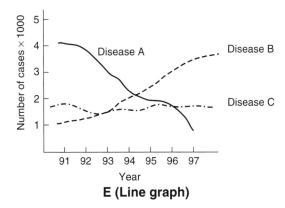

E (Line graph)

46. The answer is d. *(Rosner, 5/e, pp 9–23.)* These curves have the same mode, median, and mean (measures of location). However, the spread is different and can be assessed by computing the standard deviation (measure of dispersion), which will be different for both curves. Although a large sample size tends to reduce variation and narrow a curve, it is not a summary numerical measure.

47. The answer is b. *(Rosner, 5/e, pp 13–14.)* This curve is skewed to the *left* (or negatively skewed). Such curves have median values that are larger than the arithmetic mean, and the mean also lies to the *left* of the median. This occurs when more outlying values are smaller than the mean, or points below the median tend to be further away from the median than points above. A curve is skewed to the *right* (or positively skewed) when the opposite occurs, and the mean lies to the *right* of the median. This curve only has one mode but is not symmetrical nor normally distributed.

48–50. The answers are 48-b, 49-d, 50-a. *(Rosner, 5/e, pp 183, 239, 243–245.)* Large sample sizes increase the precision of a study and decrease the width of the confidence intervals (CI). If the confidence interval includes one when assessing relative risks or odds ratio, it includes the null value. Therefore, the *p* value will be higher than 0.05 and the study will not reach statistical significance. The smaller the sample size, the larger the CI will be, and the more likely a study will be unable to (or have the power to) demonstrate a statistical difference between two groups, and will have a "lower power." Also note that the smaller the difference between the null and alternative means, the larger the sample size will need to be in order to demonstrate a statistical difference and reject the null hypothesis.

51–53. The answers are 51-d, 52-b, 53-c. *(Rosner, 5/e, pp 63–65.)* This is an example of receiver-operator curves, or ROC curves. The horizontal axis (x) represents $1 -$ specificity, or the false-positive rate. This is plotted against the sensitivity on the vertical axis (y). There is always a trade-off between sensitivity and specificity as no test is ever 100% sensitive and 100% specific. Each curve can be used to determine the optimal cut-off point for the respective test. In general, the point closest to the upper-left corner, where sensitvity is highest and the false-positive rate is lowest, is chosen as the cut-off. The area under the curve is used to calculate the diagnostic accuracy (best combined sensitivity and specificity) of the test, that is, the probability of correctly identifying disease or no disease based on the result of the test. The larger the area under the curve, the "better" the test. In this example, test C has the largest area under the curve compared to the other tests, and therefore would have the greatest diagnostic accuracy.

54. The answer is c. *(Greenberg, 2/e, pp 161–163.)* Sensitivity analysis is used in decision analysis to determine how much impact different probabilities of a particular event will have on the choice of choosing one intervention over another. Computer programs can compute and plot these data. The maximum quality-adjusted life expectancy or years (or QALYs) for surgery is 4.5 and for radiation is 4.2. QALYs are plotted for radiation therapy and surgery for different probabilities of mortality from surgery. As expected, mortality from surgery does not impact the QALYs obtained from radiation therapy. However, as mortality from surgery increases, the QALYs for that intervention decrease. If mortality did not impact QALYs for surgery, you would obtain a straight line with the y coordinate at 4.5. The threshold is the point at which both interventions intersect: decisions will be made above or below that point. In this case, surgery is superior to radiation if the mortality is below 11%. However, if the mortality from surgery is higher than 11%, then you gain more QALYs from radiation therapy. The sensitvity analysis from this example demonstrates that mortality rate from surgery is an important variable for determining the best strategy.

55. The answer is e. *(Rosner, 5/e, pp 219, 243–244.)* The null hypothesis (the odds ratio equals one) is not rejected. The confidence interval includes 1, and the p value is higher than 0.05. There is a 95% confidence interval, so the alpha was set at 0.05. If the alpha is set at 0.10, we want to be 90% confident that the interval limits cover the true value of the odds ratio. This would therefore narrow the width of the confidence interval. Conversely, if we were to choose an alpha at 0.01, or wanting to be 99% confident that the limits cover the true value, the confidence interval would be larger.

56. The answer is c. *(Rosner, 5/e, pp 425–455, 466–487, 612–625.)* Simple linear regression examines the association between two continuous variables, the outcome/response variable *y* (the glomerular filtration rate), also called the dependent variable, and a predictor/explanatory variable *x* (the plasma creatinine), also called the independent variable. The line $y = \alpha + \beta x$ expresses the relationship and is called the regression line where alpha is the intercept and beta the slope. The ultimate objective is to predict the value of an outcome based on the fixed value of an explanatory variable. In this example, we would be able to predict the glomerular filtration rate from a particular value of plasma creatinine, and thus determine what is considered to be within normal limits. Multiple regression is used when we wish to examine the relationship between multiple dependant variables and the independent variable. The relationship is expressed as $y = \alpha + \beta_1 x_1 + \beta_{2x2} + \cdots + \varepsilon$. Logistic regression is used when *y* (the dependent variable) is not a continuous variable, but rather a dichotomous variable (for example, presence or absence of disease). The goal would then be to predict the presence or absence of disease based on a certain value of

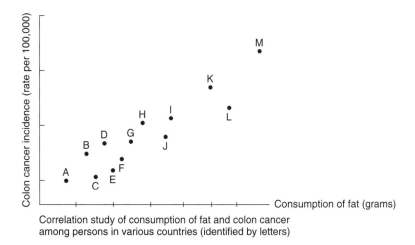

Correlation study of consumption of fat and colon cancer
among persons in various countries (identified by letters)

the predictor variable. Correlation analysis is used to determine whether there is a *linear* relationship between continuous variables that are treated symmetrically. It would not identify relationships that are nonlinear. It does not imply a cause and effect relationship, nor does it describe the nature of the relationship. It is used to analyze relationships in correlation studies of population. Is there a linear relationship between fat consumption and colon cancer, immunization rates and infant mortality? Each country represents a point in the plot with a combination of outcomes x,y.

57. The answer is d. *(Greenberg, 3/e, pp 112–115.)* Both studies have the same relative risk (0.6/1.3 and 9.2/20 = 0.46). The intervention reduces the mortality by more than 50%. The relative risk reduction is expressed as risk of mortality in the intervention group (RI) − risk of mortality in the control group (RC)/RC. For study A: |0.6 − 1.3|/1.3 = 0.54 and for study B: |9.2 − 20|/20 = 0.54. It represents the *proportional* reduction in rates of a "bad" event between the intervention group and the control group, and basically gives similar information as the relative risk. These two measures are useful to determine the magnitude of the effect of a given intervention. These measures can be misleading in assessing the clinical relevance of an intervetion because the overall impact of the intervention is highly dependent on the rate of mortality in the control. In study A, the rate in the control group is very low. Thus, even if the relative risk is very high, the intervention is associated with little overall gain. The absolute risk reduction (ARR) is expressed as RI − RC. It is the arithmetic difference between the two groups, or the same as attributable risk. We say *reduction* if the intervention reduces the risk and *increase* if the intervention increases a particular risk (not meaning a bad outcome). For study A, the ARR is equal to a reduction of 0.7%, and for study B, it is equal to a reduction of 10.8%. This measure gives a better picture of the impact of an intervention and how much benefit can be attributed to the intervention. We can see that the intervention used in study B would provide more benefit than the intervention used in study A. Numbers needed to treat (NNT) are expressed as 1/ARR. This gives us an estimate of how many patients will need the intervention before we can avoid one bad outcome, and can be useful for clinicians to get a perspective on the intervention in their practices.

58. The answer is c. *(Rosner, 5/e, pp 603–605, 592–594.)* Since the crude and the gender-adjusted relative risks are the same, you can conclude that gender is not a confounder (using the "change-in-estimate" definition of confounding). However, the relative risk for men is different than for women. We conclude that gender is an effect modifier. Effect modification is a different concept than confounding. *Confounding* is a "nuisance" factor that needs to be eliminated because it causes a distortion of the results, simply because that factor is distributed unevenly in exposed and unexposed individuals. Effect modification provides important information: the magnitude of the effect of a particular exposure on the outcome will vary according to the presence of a third factor, in this case, gender. It is not related to the fact that there may be more men than women in one group or another. A third factor can be both a confounder and an effect modifier if the adjusted risk differs from the crude, in addition to having different risks in women and in men. It may be neither a confounder nor an effect modifer if the adjusted and crude risks are the same and if the rates in men and women were the same. Finally, it could be only a confounder if the crude and adjusted risks differ, but the rates between men and women are the same. Stratification can be used to evaluate both confounding and effect modification: it will eliminate confounding and describe effect modification.

59. The answer is a. (*Rosner, 5/e, pp 407–411.*) The Kappa statistic is often used for reliability studies. For example, it can be used to assess interrater reliability, such as comparing the readings of mammography between different radiologists. It could also be used to assess intrarater reliability, such as comparing responses from participants on surveys given more than once over a period of time to evaluate reproducibility of responses. The chi-square will not give the degree of association and is used for categorical data. The student *t* test and correlation studies are used to analyze continuous data.

60. The answer is b. (*Rosner, 5/e, p 349.*) The Wilcoxon rank sum test as well as the Wilcoxon signed rank test and the signed tests can be used when we cannot assume that the underlying population is of normal distribution, especially when dealing with small samples. The signed test and the signed rank tests are the counterparts (for nonparametric distributions) of the paired *t* test, and the rank sum is analoguous to the *t* test for independent samples. A drawback of nonparametric methods is that they have less power than the methods used when normal distribution is assumed. The chi-square test is used for categorical data. The Mantel-Haenszel is a statistical method used to control for confounding. Analysis of variance is used to test the difference between the means of more than two independent samples.

61. The answer is b. *(Greenberg, 2/e, pp 18–19. Hennekens and Buring, pp 64–66.)* Prevalence is equal to incidence times the duration of disease, or $P = I \times D$. The longer the duration of the disease, the more likely it is to be present at any given time. If a disease has a high mortality rate (short duration), it is unlikely to be counted at any time. Prevalence of disease will increase when a new treatment decreases mortality. A high incidence of disease may or may not have an impact on prevalence: it will depend on its duration and mortality rate.

62. The answer is a. *(Pagano, p 314.)* The degrees of freedom for the chi-square distribution are calculated as follows: (rows − 1)(columns − 1). So, for a contingency table as the one illustrated 2×2, the degrees of freedom would be $(2 - 1)(2 - 1) = 1$. If we were using a 3×4 table, then the degrees of freedom would be $(3 - 1)(4 - 1) = 6$.

63. The answer is c. *(Greenberg, 2/e, pp 2–22. Rosner, 5/e, pp 713–716.)* This is an example of a Kaplan-Meier method, also called the product-limit method, of estimating survival. This technique takes into consideration that not all individuals may be followed until they experience the end point or "failure" (in this example, death). Some may be lost to follow-up prior to failure (move away, refuse to continue to participte any longer, etc.), and others who have not experienced an end point may not have been followed for the *whole* observation period because they entered late in the course of the study. These are called *censored observations* (incomplete observation of a time to failure). Kaplan-Meier curves appear like uneven steps. Other methods can be used (actuarial method), but the Kaplan-Meier is the most frequent.

64–67. The answers are 64-d, 65-c, 66-b, 67-e. *(Wallace, 14/e, p 49.)* Fetal mortality is defined as the number of stillbirths per 1000 births of gestational age greater than 28 weeks. It evaluates fetal losses of the third trimester. Maternal mortality refers to the death of a woman from *any* cause *related to or aggravated by* pregnancy or its management. *Direct* maternal mortality relates to the death of a woman from obstetrical complications of pregnancy, labor, puerperium, from interventions, omissions, or treatment (such uterine rupture, prolapse, etc.). *Indirect* maternal mortality relates to conditions aggravated or caused by pregnancy, labor, or puerperium (diabetes, congenital heart disease, etc.) but not directly obstetrical.

68–69. The answers are 68-b, 69-c. *(Greenberg et al., 2/e, pp 133–135.)* Internal validity can be questioned if there is systematic (nonrandom) error in the way information is collected. Systematic errors include bias and confounding. If a study suffers from lack of internal validity due to serious selection or information bias, and/or failure to control for confounding, the results should be questioned. External validity refers to whether the results (internally valid) of a study can be applied to the other populations. This is a question of judging whether the subjects in the study are similar to the population you are interested in applying the results to (such as patients in your clinical practice). Power refers to the capability of a study to detect statistically significant results. Reliability is synonymous with precision: even though the results in the study described in question 69 reached statistical significance (the CI does not include 1), there is a very large confidence interval, suggesting that the study is not precise (increased random error). Lack of precision is often due to small sample sizes.

70–73. The answers are 70-b, 71-a, 72-d, 73-c. *(Rosner, 5/e, pp 776–779.)* Use of the student *t* test to assess the difference between the mean systolic pressures of pregnant and nonpregnant women would be appropriate since the two groups are independent samples and the outcome variable is quantitative (continuous) and approximately normally distributed.

In the study comparing the occurrence of hepatitis B surface antigen in medical and dental students, use of chi-square analysis would be appropriate because both the predictor and outcome variables are categorical and dichotomous; that is, students are classified by the presence or absence of the antigen and by medical or dental student status. The McNemar test is used for a matched pair of categorical data.

To compare the levels of blood glucose in rats to whom a drug was administered, analysis of variance would be appropriate because six different groups are to be analyzed (two sexes and three drugs), where one variable is categorical (sex/drug) and the other is continuous (glucose level). Analysis of variance will permit evaluation of the effects and interaction of sex and drug on the glucose level.

The paired *t* test is appropriate for comparing paired (e.g., before and after) measurements. Use of the regular (student two-sample) *t* test in this instance is inappropriate because the two samples are not independent—the same subjects are in each.

74–77. The answers are 74-b, 75-a, 76-e, 77-f. (*Greenberg, 2/e, pp 80–81, 139–143.*) Effect modification occurs when one factor modifies the effect on outcome of another. As an example, a high bilirubin seems to be a much stronger risk factor for bilirubin-induced brain damage if the baby is sick in other ways (see question 58.)

Confounding occurs when the association between two variables is distorted by the fact that both are associated with a third. For example, the association between coffee and lung cancer is distorted by smoking: among nonsmokers and smokers considered separately, coffee and lung cancer may be completely unrelated, but when the two groups are combined, an association appears to be present. Similarly, lead levels need to be related to IQ separately at each level of socioeconomic status to assure that the association is not due to confounding. The possibility that hyperactive children have high lead levels because they are hyperactive, rather than vice versa, is not confounding; it is simply a case in which the direction of causality is turned around (effect-cause). Nondifferential misclassification results in the mixing of two groups because the measure of either the exposure or the outcome was imprecise, for example, assessing precise diet habits by questionnaires in a case-control study, and going back many years. Most people are unlikely to remember what and how much they ate years ago, and thus exposures will be similar in the cases and controls. Recall bias, a form of differential misclassification, is unlikely in this setting. *Nondifferential misclassification always biases results toward the null value.*

Lead-time bias refers to a distortion of the apparent efficacy of a screening program (see answer to question 16).

78–81. The answers are 78-a, 79-c, 80-b, 81-e. (*Greenberg, 2/e, pp 15–19, 113.*) The *point prevalence* is the proportion of people in a population who have a disease at a given point in time. The numerator is the number of existing cases of a disease; the denominator is the total population at risk of the disease at that point in time.

In order to compare rates of disease or death in two or more groups that differ substantially in age, sex, or racial composition, adjustment or standardization of the rates is necessary to remove the effects of those differences. The *standardized mortality or morbidity ratio* (SMR) is the ratio of the observed number to the expected number of deaths or cases of the disease. For example, age-specific rates of angina pectoris in nonsmokers can be applied to the age distribution of smokers to obtain the expected number of cases of angina pectoris in the smokers. The SMR of smokers for angina pectoris is the observed number of cases divided by the expected number so calculated.

The *cumulative incidence* is the number of new cases of a disease that occur in a period of time divided by the population at risk during that time. The incidence density takes into consideration the length of time subjects participated in the study and the denominator is expressed in person-time of observation.

The relative risk (or risk ratio) is the incidence of disease in subjects with a risk factor divided by the incidence in those in whom the factor is absent. (The denominator is not the incidence in the general population because then subjects with the risk factor would be included. If the risk factor is uncommon and the relative risk is close to 1.0, the error involved in using the general population for the denominator is small. However, other risk factors, for instance, a relative with CHD, are quite prevalent.) The term *relative risk* can be confusing when the risk factor has to do with being a relative of a patient; in this instance, *risk ratio* is a preferable synonym.

82–86. The answers are 82-c, 83-e, 84-d, 85-b, 86-a. (*Greenberg, 2/e, pp 80–82. Rosner, 5/e, pp 212–216.*) Although these terms are usually applied to epidemiological studies, they are also applicable to examples from everyday life. *Lead-time bias* commonly refers to the apparent increase in life expectancy seen in patients who have their disease diagnosed with a screening test. The problem is that the screening test does not actually result in the patients' living any longer than they would have otherwise; the fact is simply that these patients are detected with the disease earlier in the disease's course. The same would be true of a study that found that anatomy students lived at the same address for a longer period of time than fourth-year medical students, most of whom move to start internships. The study would not be wrong, but any conclusions that suggested that anatomy students are more stable than fourth-year clerks would be meaningless.

Surveillance bias refers to overdetection of the disease of interest because one of the groups goes to the doctor (or has a diagnostic test) more often than does another group. Similarly, you are more likely to find something that is lost in June (when you may be moving) than in March, when you are presumably in the middle of the term.

Recall bias classically refers to a situation in which persons with a disease are more likely to remember an exposure (say, to a toxic chemical) than persons who are healthy. This is part of a human tendency to look for explanations for bad outcomes—like failing an examination.

A type 1 error occurs when a result is found to be statistically significant by chance in a sample even though there is no effect in the population. In the case of answering the question correctly, the chance of a type 1 error is 20% because even if you did not know anything about this question, you would have a 1 in 5 chance of getting it correct.

Power is the chance of finding an effect in your sample if it truly exists in the population. One problem with finding out that your friends have been out at the movies is that they may not tell you the truth (recall bias), or you may ask the wrong ones, such as those sitting next to you in the library (surveillance bias). So you can give yourself credit if you made one of those choices as well, assuming you understood what you were doing!

87–90. The answers are 87-b, 88-e, 89-a, 90-c. (Greenberg, pp 22–23, 49–53.) The case fatality rate is a measure of the severity of the disease. It is a ratio of the number of deaths caused by a disease to the total number of cases of that disease and is usually expressed as a percentage. The crude mortality equals the total number of deaths from all causes during a year divided by the average population at risk during that year. It is usually expressed as the number of deaths per 1000 people. The secondary attack rate is a measure of the contagiousness of an infectious disease. The numerator is the number of cases of disease in contacts of the index case; the denominator is the number of contacts exposed to the index case during a specified period. Rates of disease are called morbidity rates.

91–94. The answers are 91-b, 92-a, 93-e, 94-b. (Greenberg, 2/e, pp 19–21, 125. Rosner, 5/e, pp 591–596.) Matching is a way of selecting subjects that are comparable with respect to specific variables. For example, in a case-control study, a control could be selected that is the same age and sex as the case. It is thus a sampling strategy to achieve comparability among groups.

Stratification is an analysis strategy with the same purpose. Thus, after the study has been completed, the subjects can be stratified, that is, divided into separate, relatively homogeneous strata, and the comparison between groups can occur within each stratum. For example, survival could be compared separately in different age strata, as in question 91. This might be important if the subjects with high renin levels were also older than the subjects with low levels, since a difference in survival between the two groups might be due to age, rather than to differing renin levels.

Age adjustment takes stratification by age one step further. After mortality (or another parameter) is calculated for specific age strata, it is combined in a weighted average to yield a single number. The weights used are the sizes of the different age strata in a standard population. Age adjustment is used more often for comparing mortality in populations with differing age structures.

Multivariate statistical analysis, like stratification, is an analysis technique for achieving comparability among groups. It involves modeling the associations between variables in order to allow their different effects to be isolated from each other. (For example, in multiple regression, the relationships between variables are modeled as a straight line.)

Survival analysis is a technique by which persons followed for variable lengths of time are counted according to the length of time they were followed. For example, in the cohort study of renin levels mentioned previously, instead of simply comparing the proportions surviving five years, the cumulative probability of survival could be plotted for the two groups, and the two curves compared. The Kaplan-Meier and life table analysis are two methods used for survival analysis. The first plots the percentage of persons alive after each year since a diagnosis.

95–98. The answers are 95-d, 96-a, 97-b, 98-d. *(Hennekens, pp 58, 132, 170.)* For proper comparison of the frequency of a disease in two groups, the rate of disease, not the number of cases, must be compared. The number of cases may reflect the age structure of the population served by the hospital. Age-specific attack rates that incorporate the number of cases in each age group, divided by the number of persons in each group, should be calculated.

In order to determine that an association between two conditions such as diabetes and obesity exists, an investigator must show that obesity is significantly more common in persons who have diabetes than in persons who do not have diabetes. The controls are necessary in order to test the significance of the association and must resemble the cases as closely as possible in all ways except for the absence of the disease under study.

Whenever considerable numbers of a cohort are lost to follow-up, doubts about the validity of the conclusions arise. Because death may be a major reason for loss to follow-up, the most conservative approach is to assume that everyone lost to follow-up has died. Unless, in this example, the death rate in the anxiety neurosis cohort was still no greater than that in the general population (after adding another 50 deaths for the 20% of the 250 patients lost to follow-up), the conclusions are suspect.

The conclusion in question 98 is invalid because of the lack of denominators to calculate the rate of bacterial endocarditis in different age groups. In addition, the autopsy series merely gives an estimate of the proportion of deaths in different age groups, not the frequency of occurrence of endocarditis with age. The autopsy series may also be invalid as a source of data from which to draw conclusions because of factors that determined whether an autopsy was performed.

99–102. The answers are 99-b, 100-c, 101-a, 102-e. *(Greenberg, 2/e, pp 159–164.)* When constructing a decision analysis tree, the first node is a decision node to reflect the choices you have to make to manage a specific medical problem. Branches from the chance nodes must reflect all possibilities. Terminal nodes reflect the outcomes or utilities assigned to the outcomes, such as death, survival, quality-adjusted life years, and so forth. The tree is "folded back" from right to left to get the expected utilities for each choice of action. Thus, the utilities are expressed in the same units as the outcomes (e.g., probability of survival, quality-adjusted life years). Here, the utility for surgery is equal to $(0 \times 0.05) + \{[(4.4 \times 0.05) + (4.8 \times 0.95)] \times 0.95\} = 4.5$. Therefore, surgery provides more QALYs than radiation therapy. If radiation therapy was never associated with proctitis, then you use the QALYs associated with the branch "no proctitis," $(3.5 \times 0.40) + (5.0 \times 0.60) \times 1.0 = 4.4$

103–106. The answers are 103-a, 104-d, 105-e, 106-c. *(Hennekens, pp 73–88.)* If the probability of an event is p, the odds of the event are $p / (1 - p)$. The odds ratio is the ratio of the odds of exposure to the risk factor given disease (a/c) to the odds of exposure to the risk factor given no disease (b/d). To illustrate that the odds of exposure given disease are a/c, the probability of exposure given disease is $5a/(a + c)$. So $(1 - p) = c/(a + c)$, and the odds are $[a/(a + c)]/[c/(a + c)]$, and the $(a + c)$ phrases cancel out to give a/c. The odds ratio, therefore, is $(a/c) / (b/d)$, which equals ad/bc.

Odds ratios are mainly used in case-control studies, from which relative risk cannot be calculated directly. When the disease is rare, the odds ratio closely approximates the relative risk. However, the study in the example is a cohort study, so relative risk can be calculated directly from the table. It is equal to the risk (incidence) of suicide in those who served in Vietnam divided by the risk in those who served elsewhere, or $[a/(a + b)]/[c/(c + d)]$.

Excess risk is defined as the difference between the risk in those with the risk factor and those in whom it is absent. Whereas the relative risk and odds ratio are unitless (since any measurements of time in the denominators cancel out), the excess risk must have an explicit or implied time period in the denominator. In this example, $a/(a + b) - c/(c + d)$ represents the excess risk of suicide in Vietnam veterans over a five-year period; it is five times as big as the excess risk for a one-year period. Thus, if the yearly risk of suicide was 0.2% in Vietnam veterans and 0.1% in other veterans, the relative risk would be 2.0, and the excess risk (risk difference) 0.1% per year, or 0.5% over the five-year period.

The overall incidence of suicide (per five years) in the study is simply the number of suicides $(a + c)$ divided by the population at risk $(a + b + c + d)$. (Note that a more precise way to measure the incidence, relative risk, and so on would be to use person-years at risk in the denominators, but this leads to greater computational and conceptual complexity.)

107–110. The answers are 107-c, 108-e, 109-a, 110-d. *(Pagano, pp 469–472.)* Simple random sampling is a process in which individuals are sampled independently, and each individual of the population has an equal probability of being selected.

In cluster sampling, groups of people (e.g., families, school classes) are selected at random, and then everyone in those groups is sampled. A common analytic mistake is to pretend that subjects obtained in a cluster sample were obtained in a simple random sample. This can lead to incorrect results because the subjects are not sampled independently.

Systematic sampling is a process that first requires the arrangement of the group to be sampled in some kind of order. Then individuals are selected systematically throughout the series on the basis of a predetermined sampling fraction or constant determinant, for example, every fifth, tenth, or hundredth person in the ordered group. Although systematic sampling may seem almost the same as simple random sampling, it is much less desirable. For example, sampling every other subject from a list in which husbands' and wives' names appear next to each other (e.g., an alphabetical list) will bias the sample—if husbands were always first, the sample might include no wives and would rarely include both persons in a married couple.

In stratified sampling, a population is divided into subgroups based on defined characteristics such as age, sex, or severity of illness, or any combination of these; then random samples are selected from each subgroup. For example, you could take a random sample from a group of 15- to 19-year-olds, from a group of 20- to 24-year-olds and from a group of 25- to 29-year-olds from a total population of 14- to 29-year-olds. This is used particularly in situations where the distribution of each subgroup is not uniform in the group as a whole (for instance, there may be only a few 14- to 15-year-olds, and they may be missed if you were to use a simple random sample of the 14- to 29-year-old group). This method allows you to make sure that persons from each subgroup are represented in your sample.

In paired sampling, or matching, selection of one or more controls for each case is based on age, sex, time, time sequence, geographic location, or some other defined relationship to the case (so it is not random). For example, selection could be based on the next patient admitted after each case, the sibling nearest in age to each case, or the person who lives closest geographically to each case.

111–115. The answers are 111-d, 112-c, 113-a, 114-b, 115-e.
(*Greenberg, 2/e, pp 76–81.*) The easiest (and best) way to answer problems like this is to write out the appropriate 2 × 2 table. Since we were not told how many women were tested, we can just make up a number—say, 200. We are told that half have a positive test:

	Infection	No Infection	
Test positive	?	?	100
Test negative	?	?	100
			200

The next task is to fill in the remaining boxes. We are told that 45% of those with a positive test are infected with chlamydia:

	Infection	No Infection	
Test positive	45	55	100
Test negative	?	?	100
			200

and that 95% of those with a negative test are free of the disease:

	Infection	No Infection	
Test positive	45	55	100
Test negative	5	95	100
	50	150	200

This now allows us to say that for 200 women in the community, the following 2 × 2 table would be correct:

	Infection	No Infection	
Test positive	45	55	100
Test negative	5	95	100
	50	150	200

We can now determine the test's operating characteristics (sensitivity and specificity) and the other parameters. Sensitivity is simply the proportion of women with chlamydia who will have a positive test (remember: PID = positive in disease), or 45/50 = 90%. Specificity is the proportion of women without chlamydia who will have a negative test (remember: NIH = negative in health), or 95/150 = 63%. The prevalence of the disease is simply the proportion of women with chlamydia, or 50 out of 200 = 25%. The predictive value of a positive test is the proportion of women with a positive test who have chlamydia; we were already told that this was 45%. Likewise, the predictive value of a negative test is the proportion of women with a negative test who do not have chlamydia; we were already told that this was 95%.

116–119. The answers are 116-c, 117-a, 118-b, 119-d. *(Greenberg, 2/e, pp 123–125, 175. Rosner, 5/e, pp 213–215. Pagano, pp 218–222.)* A type 2 error occurs when a study fails to reject the null hypothesis (of no effect) when it is in fact false. Any time a study fails to achieve statistical significance, a crucial question to ask is whether the study had enough subjects. Although 500 subjects per group followed for five years seems like a large number, only a tiny minority (perhaps 10 per group) would be expected to have a myocardial infarction. Thus, the sample size in this instance may have been inadequate to detect a meaningful difference between the groups.

The ecologic fallacy occurs when associations among groups of subjects are mistakenly assumed to hold for individuals. Thus, although among communities, high rates of condom use may be associated with higher fertility rates (perhaps because condom use acts as a marker for sexual activity in general), among those who use the condoms, the fertility rate could in fact be zero.

A type 1 error occurs when, just by chance, a statistically significant difference between groups is found. Studies attempting to correlate multiple risk factors with multiple diseases (particularly when there is no good biologic reason to suspect an association) are especially prone to type 1 errors. Looking for associations separately in different subgroups compounds the problem.

Selection bias occurs when the subjects selected for the study are somehow not representative of the population from which they come. One trouble with selecting spouses for controls is that one's spouse is much more likely to share one's smoking habits than a person from the general population. Thus, since patients with lung cancer will be mostly smokers, smokers will be overrepresented among the controls, and smoking will look like a weaker risk factor than it really is.

120–124. The answers are 120-a, 121-c, 122-e, 123-b, 124-d. (*Pagano, pp 7–11.*) The scale of measurement is an important determinant of the amount of information in a variable and the type of statistical analysis that can be used. Dichotomous variables (like sex) have only two possible values. Some variables may be artificially dichotomized, with subsequent loss of information. For example, a patient either survives five years or not; thus survival to five years is an example of a dichotomous variable. The variable could be made more informative, however, if the actual number of months of survival was specified.

Nominal variables have more than two possible values, but no intrinsic ordering. Race is the classic example; medical specialties also have no intrinsic ordering. Nominal and ordinal are often confused. Just remember *nominal* for "no ordering."

Ordinal variables are intrinsically ordered, but not in a quantitative way that allows one to say that there is a natural numerical distance between possible values. Thus, one value cannot really be subtracted from another. Examples are qualitative judgments such as "worse, same, better" or "never, sometimes, always." Remember, *ordinal* means "ordered."

Interval scales are ordered, but with real numerical units; they can be subtracted from each other. An example is dates of birth: they are intrinsically ordered and subtracting them gives meaningful numbers, but there is no intrinsic zero to the scale, so that dividing them does not make sense— one date of birth cannot be twice as big as another.

Ratio scales are measurements in relation to a clear zero point. Thus, measurements on ratio scales can be meaningfully divided by each other. For example, one baby may weigh twice as much as another or have twice as high a platelet count. Absolute temperature is measured on a ratio scale, whereas temperature in Fahrenheit or Celsius is measured on an interval scale.

125–127. The answers are 125-a, 126-b, 127-e. (*USPS Task Force, 2/e, pp xliii–xliv.*) Answering the first two of these questions is easiest if the results of Dr. Blues's research are displayed in a 2 × 2 table:

	Depressed	**Not Depressed**
Positive Blues test	80	60
Negative Blues test	20	340
Total	100	400

The sensitivity of a test is defined as the proportion of persons with a disease who have a positive test (positive in disease = PID): in this case, 80 out of 100, or 80%. This is the same as the likelihood that a person with depression will have a positive Blues test. The specificity of a test is defined as the proportion of persons without a disease who have a negative test (negative in health = NIH): in this case, 340 out of 400, or 85%. The likelihood that someone with a negative test will be depressed (posttest probability of disease) is surely less than the overall prevalence of depression in the population (10% = pretest probability of disease).

128–130. The answers are 128-c, 129-i, 130-j. (*Greenberg, 2/e, pp 76–78.*) The probability of a positive test is the sum of all positives, true positives (TP) and false-positives (FP). Similarly, the probability of a negative test is the sum of all negatives, true negatives (TN) and false-negatives (FN). When applied to a population, calculations can be done as follows:

True positives (TP): Sensitivity × Prevalence of disease
False-positives (FP): (1 − Specificity) × (1 − Prevalence)
True negatives (TN): Specificity × (1 − Prevalence)
False-negatives (FN): (1 − Sensitivity) × Prevalence

The probability of infection given that the test is positive is the definition of positive predictive value (PPV) and can be described as TP/(TP + FP). The probability of no infection given a positive test can be described as 1 − PPV. The probability of no infection given that the test is negative is the negative predictive value (NPV), expressed as TN/(TN + FN). The probability of infection given a negative test can be expressed as 1 − NPV. The tree can be completed as follows:

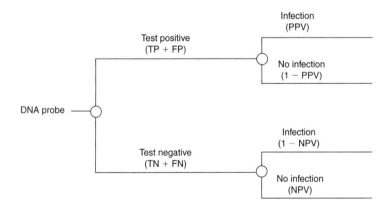

EPIDEMIOLOGY AND PREVENTION OF COMMUNICABLE DISEASES

Questions

DIRECTIONS: Each item below contains a question or incomplete statement followed by suggested responses. Select the **one best** response to each question.

131. A 6-year-old child is brought to the emergency room by her parents on a Friday night because they are concerned about rabies. A bat was present in the child's bedroom when they arrived at their country home that evening. It started flying around the head of the girl when she entered her room and it ruffled her hair. The parents heard her scream, ran up to her room, and shooed the bat out the window. Upon examination, there is no visible bite or scratch marks. Which is the most appropriate intervention at this time?

a. Reassure the parents that there is no risk of rabies given the history and examination
b. Consult public health authorities to determine the epidemiology of rabies in that area
c. Administer rabies vaccine and rabies immunoglobulin (RIG)
d. Administer rabies immunoglobulin (RIG) only
e. Administer rabies vaccine only

132. Which of the following conditions has been associated with a false-positive Fluorescent Treponemal Antibody Absorption (FTA-ABS) test?

a. Tuberculosis
b. Mononucleosis
c. Lyme disease
d. Viral pneumonia
e. HIV infection

133. One of your patients, a 30-year-old developer, tells you he is planning a trip to the Dominican Republic the following month. He will need to travel in rural areas. Which is the most appropriate intervention for malaria prophylaxis for this patient?

a. No prophylaxis
b. Chloroquine
c. Mefloquine
d. Doxycycline
e. Primaquine

134. A 20-month-old child presents to your office with a mild viral infection. The results of examination are normal except for a temperature of 37.2°C (99°F) and clear nasal discharge. Review of her vaccination records reveals that she received only two doses of polio vaccine and diphtheria-tetanus-pertussis (DTaP) vaccine, and that she did not receive the measles-mumps-rubella (MMR) vaccine. The mother is 20 weeks pregnant. Her brother is undergoing chemotherapy for leukemia. Which of the following is the most appropriate intervention?

a. Schedule a visit in two weeks for DTaP
b. Administer inactivated polio vaccine (IPV) and DTaP
c. Administer DTaP, oral polio vaccine (OPV), and MMR
d. Administer DTaP, IPV, and MMR
e. Administer DTaP and OPV and schedule a visit in three months for MMR

135. Prevention of human brucellosis depends primarily on

a. Pasteurization of dairy products derived from goats, sheep, or cows
b. Treatment of human cases
c. Control of the insect vector
d. Immunization of farmers and slaughterhouse workers
e. Destruction of infected animals

136. Which of the following vaccines is CONTRAINDICATED during pregnancy?

a. Hepatitis B vaccine
b. Varicella vaccine
c. Influenza vaccine
d. Tetanus toxoid
e. Rabies vaccine

137. A 32-year-old farmer presents to the emergency room with a crushing injury of the index finger and thumb that occurred while he was working with machinery in his barn. Records show that he received three doses of Td in the past, and that his last dose was given when he was 25 years old. In addition to proper wound cleaning and management, which of the following is the most appropriate prevention intervention?

a. No additional prophylaxis
b. Administration of tetanus toxoid
c. Administration of tetanus immunoglobulin only
d. Administration of tetanus toxoid and immunoglobulin
e. Administration of tetanus and diphtheria toxoid

138. Epidemics of typhus fever have been associated with war and famine for several centuries. What factor was most important in the control of such epidemics following the end of World War II?

a. Eradication of *Anopheles* mosquitoes
b. Improved sanitation practices
c. Improved methods for handling food supplies
d. Disinfestation by use of DDT
e. Mass therapy with antibiotics

139. Immunization of preschool children with diphtheria toxoid results in

a. Protection against the diphtheria carrier state
b. Lifelong immunity against diphtheria
c. Detectable antitoxin or immunologic memory for about 10 years
d. Frequent adverse reactions
e. Protection against infection of the respiratory tract by *Corynebacterium diphtheriae*

140. What is the recommended interval in months between the administration of whole blood transfusion and the measles-mumps-rubella (MMR) vaccine?

a. 0
b. 1
c. 3
d. 6
e. 10

141. Professional organizations recommend that all pregnant women be routinely counseled about HIV infection and be encouraged to be tested. What is the most important reason for early identification of HIV infection in pregnant women?

a. A cesarean section can be planned to reduce HIV transmission to the newborn
b. Breast feeding can be discouraged to reduce transmission to the newborn
c. Early identification of a newborn at risk of HIV infection will improve survival
d. Counseling on pregnancy options, such as termination, can be offered
e. Antiretroviral therapy can be offered to reduce the chance of transmission of HIV to the newborn

142. A 35-year-old patient comes to your office in early April for a routine examination. In the course of the history, he tells you that he plans to go turkey hunting in Nantucket, Massachusetts, for one week in May. He is concerned about Lyme disease. Which is the most appropriate intervention for preventing Lyme disease?

a. Vaccination
b. Avoidance of bushy areas
c. Tick check at the end of each day
d. Protective clothing and DEET
e. Antibiotic prophylaxis for one week

Items 143–144

An 18-year-old sexually active college student presents with complaints of lower abdominal pain and irregular bleeding for five days. She has no fever. She uses oral contraceptives as method of birth control. Upon examination, the cervix is friable, there is cervical motion tenderness and adnexal tenderness. The pregnancy test is negative.

143. Which is the most likely etiologic agent responsible for these findings?

a. *Neisseria gonorrhoeae*
b. *Chlamydia trachomatis*
c. *Treponema pallidum*
d. Herpes simplex virus type 2
e. *Mycoplasma hominis*

144. She tells you that she had a similar episode two years ago. What is her risk of infertility following this second clinical episode of pelvic inflammatory disease?

a. <1%
b. 5%
c. 10%
d. 20%
e. 40%

145. In the course of investigating a 24-year-old HIV-infected male, the HBsAg is positive. He is currently asymptomatic, his physical examination is essentially normal, and his CD4 cell count is 800. Which of the following tests is most helpful in determining whether the patient is in the acute phase of viral hepatitis?

a. ALT levels
b. HBeAg
c. HBsAg
d. IgG anti-HBcAg
e. IgM anti-HBcAg

Items 146–148

You are a newly employed physician at a community hospital and have been given the responsibility of overseeing the infection control program. You plan to conduct a prospective surveillance of nosocomial infections of patients, hire infection control personnel, and begin an educational program for hospital personnel.

146. Based on national data, you expect that the incidence of nosocomial infections in your facility will be

a. <1%
b. 1 to 2%
c. 3 to 5%
d. 6 to 8%
e. 9 to 10%

147. You expect the most common site of infection to be

a. Urinary tract
b. Surgical wounds
c. Respiratory tract
d. Bloodstream
e. Gastrointestinal tract

148. The intervention most likely to decrease the transmission of nosocomial infections in your institution is

a. Adding proper ventilation systems
b. Disinfecting sheets and towels
c. Decreasing the use of indwelling catheters
d. Enforcing adherence to hand washing
e. Eliminating common sources of infection

149. In the United States, the largest proportion of tuberculosis cases occurs among

a. HIV-infected persons
b. Injecting drug users
c. Homeless persons
d. Foreign-born persons
e. Incarcerated persons

150. Which patient is most likely to become a chronic carrier following an acute episode of hepatitis B?

a. A newborn
b. A 20-year-old female following vaginal sexual transmission
c. A 50-year-old male following rectal sexual transmission with a partner positive for HBeAg
d. A 30-year-old health care worker following a percutaneous injury
e. A 40-year-old HIV-infected male with a CD4 cell count of 200

Items 151–153

A 2-year-old child is brought to the emergency room with severe prostration, a temperature of 40°C (104°F), and a few petechial lesions around the ankles. She had mild upper respiratory symptoms until her condition started deteriorating a few hours before. A Gram stain on the buffy coat of blood reveals gram-negative diplococci. Treatment is promptly initiated.

151. The case fatality rate for this clinical manifestation of disease is

a. Less than 5%
b. 5 to 15%
c. 20 to 30%
d. 40 to 50%
e. Greater than 50%

152. Compared with the general population, the risk of developing an infection among household contacts is

a. The same
b. 10 to 20 times greater
c. 50 to 100 times greater
d. 200 to 400 times greater
e. 500 to 800 times greater

153. The child had been attending a day care center. In addition to recommending close surveillance for early signs of illness, which of the following is the most appropriate management of day care contacts?

a. No further action
b. Vaccination of children only
c. Vaccination of children and adults
d. Antibiotic prophylaxis of children only
e. Antibiotic prophylaxis of adults and children

Items 154–155

A 25-year-old man presents with a single, indurated, painless ulcer on the penis that appeared two days ago. His most recent unprotected sexual contact was 21 days before. An immediate rapid plasma reagin (RPR) test is negative.

154. The most likely diagnosis is

a. Syphilis
b. Herpes
c. Chancroid
d. Lymphogranuloma venereum
e. Donovanosis (granuloma inguinale)

155. Which sexual partners should be informed of the exposure and referred for evaluation?

a. Current sexual partners only
b. Partners of within 30 days
c. Partners of within 60 days
d. Partners of within 90 days
e. Partners of within 120 days

156. A 7-year-old girl is brought to your office by her mother because of a rash that appeared three days ago. Her temperature is 37.2°C (99°F) and her face has an intense rash with a slapped-cheek appearance. The most likely etiologic agent is

a. Adenovirus
b. Rotavirus
c. Parvovirus
d. Coxsackievirus
e. Echovirus

157. To which patient would the MMR be safe to administer?

a. A 15-month-old HIV-infected child with a CD4 cell count of 700
b. A 25-year-old pregnant woman
c. A 12-year-old asthmatic on 20 mg of oral prednisone daily for the last 20 days
d. An 18-year-old with leukemia in remission whose chemotherapy was terminated 1 month ago
e. A 17-year-old with a life-threatening anaphylactic reaction to egg ingestion

Items 158–159

On a Friday afternoon, a 30-year-old nurse is brought to employee health for evaluation following a needle-stick injury that occurred at the AIDS clinic. The source patient is known to be infected with HIV and has advanced AIDS.

158. Which of the following factors carries the greatest risk for transmission of HIV to the health care worker?

a. Depth of the injury
b. Stage of illness of the source patient
c. Presence of visible blood on the needle
d. Use of gloves during the procedure
e. Entrance of the needle into a vein or artery of the source patient

159. Which is the most appropriate course of action for this health care worker?

a. Reassure her of the low risk of infection and offer no prophylaxis for HIV infection
b. Offer single-drug antiretroviral therapy
c. Offer two-drug antiretroviral therapy
d. Offer triple-drug antiviral therapy
e. Draw an HIV antibody test and refer her to the infectious disease specialist first thing Monday morning

160. A 19-year-old college student presents to the university student health center complaining of severe coughing spells for the last four days, following initial symptoms of coryza and malaise. She is afebrile. Her medical history is uneventful, and immunizations are up to date. She is a member of the basketball team. During weekends, she babysits a 10-month-old and a 2-year-old. In terms of management of contacts, which etiological agent is the most important to include in the differential diagnosis?

a. *Streptococcus pneumoniae*
b. *Mycoplasma pneumoniae*
c. *Bordetella pertussis*
d. Influenza virus
e. *Legionella pneumophila*

161. Which of the following infections is transmitted chiefly from person to person?

a. California encephalitis
b. St. Louis encephalitis
c. West Nile–like viral encephalitis
d. Meningococcal meningitis
e. Eastern Equine Encephalitis (EEE)

162. Widespread use of the *Haemophilus influenzae* type b vaccine has resulted in a dramatic decrease in the number of cases of meningitis due to this bacterium. Which agent is now the leading cause of bacterial meningitis in children in the United States?

a. *Streptococcus pneumoniae*
b. Group B *Streptococcus pyogenes* (hemolyticus)
c. Non-type-b *Haemophilus influenzae*
d. *Escherichia coli K-1*
e. *Neisseria meningitidis*

163. The medical evaluation of a 25-year-old intravenous drug user reveals elevated liver enzymes and a positive anti-HBsAg. The most likely cause of the abnormal liver profile is hepatitis

a. A
b. B
c. C
d. D
e. E

164. As an epidemiological investigation officer for the Centers for Disease Control and Prevention, you are contacted by a local health department. They inform you that a large number of persons have acquired mild symptoms of influenza despite being vaccinated for the appropriate strain being cultured. You find that the cultured strain is the same as that incorporated into the trivalent vaccine administered throughout the world. You also note that the strain had a high case fatality rate in previous epidemics in China, where most new strains are isolated and identified for vaccine preparations. The most likely explanation for the outbreak noted by the local health department is

a. Vaccine failure
b. Antigenic drift
c. Antigenic shift
d. Herd immunity
e. Incomplete immunity from previous rhinovirus infections

165. A 38-year-old HIV-infected woman presents for follow-up evaluation. She is on antiretroviral therapy. She has no complaints. Her physical examination is normal. Her PPD is reactive at 2 mm. The chest x-ray is normal. She has no history of past TB or recent known contact with infectious TB. She lives at home alone. Her CD4 + T cell count is 180/μL. Her previous count was 175/μL. Prophylaxis is most appropriate for which of the following infections?

a. *Mycobacterium avium* complex (MAC)
b. *Cryptococcus neoformans*
c. *Mycobacterium tuberculosis*
d. *Toxoplasma gondii*
e. *Pneumocystis carinii*

166. During the investigation of an outbreak of food poisoning at a summer camp, food histories were obtained from all campers as indicated in the following table. Which of the food items was probably responsible for the outbreak?

| | Proportion of Campers Who Developed Illness (Percent) | |
	Campers Who Ate	Campers Who Did Not Eat
Food	**Specified Food**	**Specified Food**
a. Hamburger	61	48
b. Potatoes	70	35
c. Ice cream	40	50
d. Chicken	73	10
e. Lemonade	20	45

167. In 1999, the majority of cumulative cases of AIDS in the United States occurred in which exposure category?

a. Men who have sex with men
b. Users of intravenous drugs
c. Women who have sex with women
d. Hemophiliacs
e. Persons who engage in heterosexual contact

168. Which of the following complications has been associated with the recall of rotavirus vaccine?

a. Guillain-Barré syndrome
b. Hemolytic anemia
c. Febrile seizures
d. Intussusception
e. Neutropenia

169. The time interval between entry of an infectious agent into a host and the onset of symptoms is called

a. The communicable period
b. The incubation period
c. The preinfectious period
d. The noncontagious period
e. The decubation period

170. An 8-year-old child is brought to the emergency room with profuse, bloody diarrhea. The symptoms started about three days ago, but gradually worsened. He has no fever. His platelet count is 40,000. The most likely source of the enteric infection is

a. Fish
b. Chicken
c. Milk
d. Eggs
e. Beef

Items 171–173

As medical director of a division of epidemiology in a state health department, you are asked to develop a hepatitis C awareness campaign. You develop a document with answers to the most frequently asked questions (FAQ) by medical providers. You follow the 1999 CDC recommendations.

171. Which group should you recommend for routine screening?

a. Pregnant women
b. Emergency medical personnel
c. Health care workers
d. Persons who ever injected illegal drugs
e. Household contacts of HCV-positive persons

172. Which test should you recommend for screening?

a. EIA for anti-HCV
b. Immunoblot assays
c. Qualitative HCV RNA
d. Quantitative HCV RNA
e. ALT levels

173. What is the most appropriate counseling message to offer to HCV-positive pregnant women?

a. Cesarian section should be performed
b. The probability of transmission to the newborn is 5%
c. Breast feeding should be discouraged
d. Infants should receive IgG at birth
e. Infants often do poorly in the first years of life

Items 174–175

You are a public health physician working at a city health department and receive a report of a case of hepatitis A virus (HAV) infection in a 32-year-old man who lives with his wife and one-year-old twins. He is a self-employed contractor who often eats on the run. His wife works part-time at a bookstore and his children attend day care. He has no history of travel, eating raw fish, or known contact with other cases of HAV infection.

174. The first step in investigating this case is to confirm the diagnosis of HAV with

a. A report of the history and examination from the treating physician
b. Stool cultures
c. Total anti-HAV antibodies
d. IgM anti-HAV
e. HAV RNA

175. The most likely source of infection is

a. A coworker
b. Food
c. His wife
d. Water
e. His children

176. A 10-year-old boy with sickle cell disease presents with headache, anorexia, and fever. He complains of pain in the right tibia and local inflammation is noted. Osteomyelitis is diagnosed. The most likely etiologic agent is

a. *Listeria*
b. *Salmonella*
c. Shigellosis
d. *Cryptosporidium*
e. *Campylobacter*

177. HSV-2 seroprevalence has increased by over 30% over the past two decades in the United States, suggesting a continuing spread of herpes. Which of the following other epidemiologic findings have been shown by recent studies?

a. Only 50% of persons with HSV-2 antibodies have been diagnosed with herpes
b. HVS-2 seropositivity correlates with viral shedding
c. Over 95% of genital infections are caused by HSV-2
d. Recurrence rates for HSV-2 are the same as for HSV-1
e. Most transmissions occur during the symptomatic phase

178. A wildlife worker presents to the emergency room because he was bitten on the hand by a raccoon while trying to capture the animal, which appeared ill. He states he received a primary course of rabies vaccination 1½ years ago when he first started his job. The wound is immediately thoroughly cleaned by the ER staff. It is small because he was wearing gloves. Which is the most appropriate intervention for rabies prevention?

a. No further prophylaxis is necessary because of the recent vaccination
b. Administer rabies immune globulin (RIG) only
c. Administer RIG and one dose of vaccine
d. Administer one dose of vaccine only
e. Administer two doses of vaccine

Items 179–180

A 5-year-old child presents to the health department clinic with fever, malaise, and a vesicular rash that started 24 hours prior. He goes to preschool. He has one sister aged 3 and his mother is 38 weeks pregnant. Both are susceptible.

179. The child is most at risk for which of the following complications?

a. Pneumonia
b. Reye's syndrome
c. Encephalitis
d. Orchitis
e. Thrombocytopenia

180. Which of the following is the most appropriate management of contacts?

a. Observation only for all contacts
b. Vaccine for the mother, sibling, and susceptible classmates
c. Immune globulin for the mother, sibling, and susceptible classmates
d. Immune globulin for the mother and vaccine for his sibling and susceptible classmates
e. Immune globulin for the mother and sibling, and vaccine for the susceptible classmates

181. Consider the clinical presentation of the newborn in the following figure.

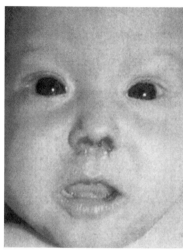

(Reproduced, with permission, from Holmes KK, Sparling PF, Mardh P, et al., *Sexually Transmitted Diseases,* 3rd ed., New York, McGraw-Hill, 1999.)

This most likely represents congenital

a. Rubella
b. Syphilis
c. Toxoplasmosis
d. Cytomegalovirus (CMV)
e. Varicella

182. Under which conditions should chemoprophylaxis for influenza be considered?

a. All nursing home residents and unvaccinated staff during an influenza A outbreak
b. All nursing home residents and unvaccinated staff during an influenza B outbreak
c. Only unvaccinated nursing home residents and staff during an influenza A outbreak
d. Only unvaccinated nursing home residents and staff during an influenza B outbreak
e. All nursing home staff and residents during an influenza B outbreak

183. For which patient is pneumococcal vaccine PPV23 not beneficial?

a. A 15-month-old HIV-infected child
b. A 20-year-old about to undergo a splenectomy for ITP
c. A 70-year-old healthy female
d. A 5-year-old with sickle cell disease
e. A 10-year-old with nephrotic syndrome who received the vaccine 5 years ago

184. Consider the epidemic curve illustrated in the following figure.

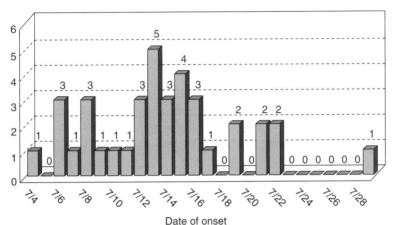

Date of onset

(*Source:* Massachusetts Department of Public Health.)

The curve most likely represents a

a. Common-source outbreak epidemic curve
b. Propagated-source outbreak epidemic curve
c. Continual-source epidemic curve
d. Person-to-person outbreak epidemic curve
e. Point-source outbreak epidemic curve

185. A 10-month-old child is brought to your office by the mother because of vomiting and profuse diarrhea for the last 24 hours. He has a temperature of 100°F and has signs of dehydration. No other person in the household is ill. The most likely etiologic agent responsible for the clinical syndrome is

a. Adenovirus
b. Rotavirus
c. Parvovirus
d. Coxsackievirus
e. Echovirus

186. The medical evaluation of a 32-year-old HIV-infected patient reveals a tuberculin skin test reaction at 5 mm. His chest x-ray is normal. He is currently taking antiretroviral therapy which includes protease inhibitors. He has not previously received therapy for tuberculosis in the past nor has he had any known contact with persons infected with tuberculosis. Which is the most appropriate intervention for this patient?

a. No preventive therapy for tuberculosis
b. Izoniazid for nine months
c. Rifampin for nine months
d. Rifampin and pyrazinamide for two months
e. Streptomycin for six months

187. HIV-infected persons are at highest risk of having an active TB infection resistant to

a. Izoniazid
b. Rifampin
c. Streptomycin
d. Ethambutol
e. Pyrazinamide

188. Four-drug therapy is recommended as an initial approach to treatment for active TB in HIV-infected persons

a. Always
b. When multidrug-resistant TB exceeds 4% in the community
c. When the patient has had previous therapy for TB
d. When the patient has had a known exposure to multi-drug resistant TB
e. When the CD4 cell count is under 200

189. You are contacted by a local physician who wishes to inform you that she diagnosed and confirmed a case of hepatitis A in one of her patients, a 5-year-old who attends a preschool center. She is concerned about the staff and children attending the school center. Which is the most appropriate management of susceptible contacts?

a. Immune globulin to all staff and children
b. Vaccine to all staff and children
c. Vaccine to staff and immune globulin to all children
d. Immune globulin and vaccine to staff and all children
e. Immune globulin only to classroom contacts

190. A 22-year-old woman presents to the obstetrical clinic for her second prenatal visit. She is 28 weeks pregnant. The examination is normal. She reports multiple sexual partners, but denies drug use. The RPR done at the first prenatal visit 8 weeks ago was 1:64 with a positive TP-PA (treponemal test). The clinic was unable to reach her. She does not recall ever being treated for syphilis in the past, nor does she remember any symptoms. The rapid RPR card test done at this visit is positive. She is allergic to penicillin. The most appropriate intervention is to

a. Send for an RPR titer and treponemal test to determine appropriate treatment
b. Treat with erythromycin
c. Treat with doxycycline
d. Admit for desensitization and treat with penicillin
e. Treat with ceftriaxone

Items 191–192

Following multiple reports of cases of *Cryptosporidium parvum* diagnosed by private physicians, as medical director of City XYZ Health Department, you conduct an epidemic investigation leading to the conclusion that the city drinking water supply is contaminated with *C. parvum*.

191. Which persons in your city are at highest risk of developing severe infection?

a. The elderly
b. Newborns and young children
c. Diabetics
d. HIV-infected persons
e. Pregnant women

192. What public health advisory measure would you announce to prevent ingestion of contaminated water?

a. Drink bottled water only
b. Use faucet filters capable of removing particles of 2.0 microns
c. Boil water for 1 minute
d. Disinfect with chlorination
e. Freeze and use thawed water

193. As medical director of a health maintenance organization, you are asked to update screening recommendations for enrolled members. You find that recommendations are lacking in the field of sexually transmitted diseases. You decide to develop evidence-based screening guidelines for *Chlamydia trachomatis*. Which of the following criteria is the most important for developing routine screening recommendations?

a. Number of sexual partners
b. Use of barrier methods such as condoms
c. Contact with an infected person
d. Presence of symptoms
e. Age

194. A 20-year-old male presents with complaints of dysuria and urethral discharge for three days. He engaged in unprotected vaginal intercourse 8 days ago with a new female sexual partner. She has no complaints. Examination reveals a yellow urethral discharge. The gram stain is as follows:

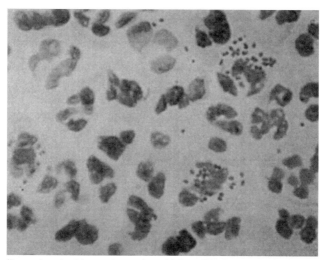

(Reproduced, with permission, from Holmes KK, Sparling PF, Mardh P, et al., *Sexually Transmitted Diseases*, 3rd ed., New York, McGraw-Hill, 1999.)

For which of the following organisms can a presumptive diagnosis be made:

a. *Chlamydia trachomatis*
b. *Treponema pallidum*
c. *Ureaplasma unrealyticum*
d. *Neisseria gonorrhoeae*
e. Herpes simplex virus infection

195. A 30-year-old Canadian immigrant farmer consults with symptoms of night sweats, low-grade fever, cough, and fatigue. He does not smoke. He has a history of asthma. The chest x-ray required for immigration was normal five months ago. He received the BCG vaccine as a child. The skin test for tuberculosis is positive at 15 mm. The most likely diagnosis is

a. Influenza
b. Brucellosis
c. Aspergillosis
d. *Mycobacterium bovis*
e. *Mycobacterium tuberculosis*

196. A healthy 2-month-old infant is brought to the office for routine child care. The child has a normal growth curve. She received the first dose of hepatitis B vaccine at birth as well as a dose of HBIG because the mother was HBsAg-positive. Which of the following vaccine series should be administered at this time?

a. MMR, OPV, DTP, Hep B
b. IPV, Hib, DTP, Hep B
c. Hep B, DTaP, Hib, IPV
d. DTaP, Hib, IPV
e. IPV, DTaP, Hep B

197. A 20-year-old college student presents to your office because she noticed two "bumps" on her vulva 1 week ago. She does not complain about pain or discharge. She has been sexually active with the same partner for one year. He has no symptoms. She has noticed one similar lesion on his penis. Upon examination, you notice two condylomata acuminata of 0.5 cm in size at the fourchette. Which of the following counseling messages is the most appropriate?

a. Treatment of her sexual partner will reduce the risk of recurrence of her vulvar lesions
b. Treatment of her vulvar lesions will reduce her risk of developing cervical cancer
c. Condom use is very effective in reducing transmission of this infection
d. Recurrence of lesions is more frequent in the first year after initial diagnosis
e. Pap smear screening should be performed every six months

DIRECTIONS: Each group of questions below consists of lettered options followed by numbered items. For each numbered item, select the appropriate lettered option(s). Each lettered option may be used once, more than once, or not at all. Choose exactly the number of options indicated following each item.

Items 198–200

Match each group of diseases with the most common described mode of transmission.

a. Water- or foodborne transmission
b. Zoonoses
c. Person-to-person direct contact transmission
d. Airborne transmission
e. Arthropod-borne transmission
f. Sexual transmission

198. Rabies, psittacosis, salmonellosis. (**SELECT 1 DESCRIPTION**)

199. Measles, tuberculosis, influenza. (**SELECT 1 DESCRIPTION**)

200. *Cyclospora, Campylobacter, Yersinia.* (**SELECT 1 DESCRIPTION**)

Items 201–204

Various terms and parameters are used in epidemiological studies of infectious diseases. Match each statement below with the most appropriate descriptive term.

a. Immunogenicity
b. Pathogenicity
c. Infectivity
d. Virulence
e. Incubation

201. Neutralizing antibody develops in 95% of people after an attack of measles. (**SELECT 1 TERM**)

202. Febrile respiratory tract disease develops in approximately 80% of children infected with influenza. (**SELECT 1 TERM**)

203. Death occurs in approximately 20% of cases of pneumococcal meningitis. (**SELECT 1 TERM**)

204. Approximately 50% of household contacts of a child who has a common cold become infected. (**SELECT 1 TERM**)

Items 205–207

Consider the epidemiologic curves of sexually transmitted diseases reported to the CDC in the United States over the last 15 years. Match each curve with the appropriate infection.

a. Chlamydia
b. Gonorrhea
c. Syphilis
d. Herpes
e. Trichomonas
f. Human papillomavirus infection
g. Hepatitis B

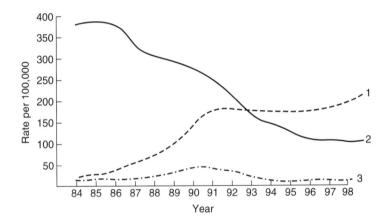

205. Curve 1

206. Curve 2

207. Curve 3

Items 208–210

Choose the most likely infectious agent for each description of the events following consumption of food.

a. Staphylococcal enterotoxin
b. *Clostridium botulinum* toxin
c. Enterotoxic *Escherichia coli*
d. *Clostridium perfringens*
e. *Salmonella typhimurium*
f. *Giardia lamblia*
g. Crytosporidium
h. Campylobacter

208. Within 4 h after attending a church supper, 25 persons report the abrupt onset of nausea, vomiting, and diarrhea. (**SELECT 1 AGENT**)

209. One week after arriving in Africa, 16 students develop vomiting, severe diarrhea, and abdominal cramps lasting 2 to 3 days. (**SELECT 1 AGENT**)

210. One-third of the persons who attended a school banquet develop abdominal cramps and watery diarrhea 8 to 12 h later. These symptoms end within 24 h. (**SELECT 1 AGENT**)

Items 211–213

Match each of the statements below with the hepatitis virus with which it has been most closely associated.

a. Hepatitis A virus (HAV)
b. Hepatitis B virus (HBV)
c. Hepatitis C virus (HCV)
d. Hepatitis D virus (HDV)
e. Hepatitis E virus (HEV)

211. Case fatality rate can be as high as 20% if acute infection occurs during the third trimester of pregnancy. (**SELECT 1 VIRUS**)

212. Coinfection must exist for replication and infection to occur. (**SELECT 1 VIRUS**)

213. Chronic disease develops in over 50% of persons following an acute infection. (**SELECT 1 VIRUS**)

Items 214–216

Match each of the diseases below with the appropriate epidemiologic term.

a. Hyperendemic
b. Epidemic
c. Endemic
d. Enzootic
e. Pandemic
f. Epizootic

214. Lyme disease in the 1990s.

215. Cholera among Rwandan refugees in 1994.

216. Influenza in 1919.

Items 217–219

Match each infection below with the intermediate host involved in transmission.

a. Snail
b. Swine
c. Fish
d. Crab
e. Dog
f. Cattle
g. Deer
h. Sheep

217. Paragonimiasis (lung fluke disease). **(SELECT 1 HOST)**

218. Toxocariasis (visceral larva migrans). **(SELECT 1 HOST)**

219. Cysticercosis. **(SELECT 1 HOST)**

Items 220–224

Select the reservoir for each of the diseases below.

a. Cattle
b. Humans
c. Rodents
d. Ticks
e. Mosquitoes
f. Cats
g. Soil
h. Vegetation

220. Nocardiosis. **(SELECT 1 RESERVOIR)**

221. Hantavirus. **(SELECT 1 RESERVOIR)**

222. Brucellosis. **(SELECT 1 RESERVOIR)**

223. Enterobiasis. **(SELECT 1 RESERVOIR)**

224. Toxoplasmosis. **(SELECT 1 RESERVOIR)**

Items 225–227

For each disease, choose the most effective or principal means of control.

a. Rat control
b. Sanitation
c. Immunization
d. Vector control
e. Deer control

225. St. Louis encephalitis. (SELECT 1 CONTROL)

226. Typhoid fever. (SELECT 1 CONTROL)

227. Tetanus. (SELECT 1 CONTROL)

Items 228–230

Match each of the descriptions below with the correct etiologic agent.

a. *Clostridium botulinum*
b. *Clostridium tetani*
c. *Poliovirus*
d. *Corynebacterium diphtheriae*
e. *Haemophilus influenza B*
f. *Borrelia burgdorferi*

228. A 25-year-old man presents with blurred vision, dysphagia, and dry mouth. (SELECT 1 AGENT)

229. A 4-year-old girl presents with sore throat, fever, hoarseness, and drooling. (SELECT 1 AGENT)

230. A 35-year-old woman presents with painful muscular contractions of the masseter and neck muscles. (SELECT 1 AGENT)

Items 231–232

For each dose schedule, select the appropriate vaccine.

a. Pneumococcal vaccine
b. Oral polio vaccine (OPV)
c. Inactivated polio vaccine (IPV)
d. Varicella vaccine
e. Measles-mumps-rubella vaccine (MMR)
f. Influenza virus vaccine

231. Recommended for the first two doses at 2 and 4 months of age.

232. Second dose recommended at age 4 to 6 years.

EPIDEMIOLOGY AND PREVENTION OF COMMUNICABLE DISEASES

Answers

131. The answer is c. *(CDC, MMWR 48[RR-1]: 8, 1999.)* Postexposure prophylaxis is recommended for *any* physical contact with bats. Bites or scratches may be too small to be visible to the naked eye. Both human rabies immunoglobulin (RIG) and vaccine should be administered to persons who have not been previously vaccinated. RIG is never recommended as only prophylaxis. It provides rapid passive protection with a half-life of 21 days. Active immunization induces response after 7 to 10 days and persists for at least 2 years. Only the vaccine is necessary if the person has a history of previous vaccination with documented antibody response. Consulting public health authorities before an intervention may be appropriate if the contact did not involve animals known to be a reservoir for rabies. Animals known to be reservoirs are the bat, skunk, raccoon, fox, coyote, and other wild carnivores, and prophylaxis is indicated regardless of the region.

132. The answer is c. *(Holmes, 3/e, p 489.)* Lyme disease (caused by *Borrelia burgdorferi,* a spirochete) has been associated with false-positive treponemal FTA-ABS (Fluorescent Treponemal Antibody Absorption) tests which are designed for the diagnosis of *Treponema pallidum* infections (i.e., syphilis). The *nontreponemal* test is often negative in this disease. Other conditions associated with false-positive *treponemal* tests include yaws, pinta, leptospirosis, and lupus. Biological false-positive *nontreponemal* tests VDRL (Venereal Disease Research Laboratory), and RPR (Rapid Plasma Reagin) are classified as acute (reverting back to negative in six months) or chronic. Acute reactions can occur with recent immunization, mononucleosis, viral pneumonia, tuberculosis, malaria, and a variety of viral diseases. Chronic reactions can occur in users of intravenous drugs, with aging, and in autoimmune diseases, such as systemic lupus erythematosus. A positive nontreponemal test must always be confirmed by a treponemal test: the

TP-PA (Treponemal Particle Absorption test) or the FTA-ABS. Nontreponemal and treponemal tests are reliable indicators of syphilis in HIV-infected persons. Although no false-positives are associated with the disease, some false-negatives may occur during end-stage disease because of severe immunosuppression.

133. The answer is b. *(Chin, 17/e, p 318.)* The Dominican Republic is one area of high risk for malaria where no chloroquine-resistant strains of *Plasmodium falciparum* have been identified. Other areas include Central America west of the Panama Canal Zone, Haiti, Egypt, and most of the Middle East. Almost all other countries with a high risk for malaria have resistant strains. The drug of choice for prophylaxis in these areas is mefloquine or doxycycline. Primaquine is given to prevent relapses due to *P. vivax* or *P. ovale*. Current information on the foci of drug-resistant *P. falciparum* is available through the Centers for Disease Control (CDC) travel Web site or the annual publication of the World Health Organization (WHO).

134. The answer is d. *(Chin, 17/e, p 402.)* Children who are late in their immunization schedule should be vaccinated when the opportunity arises. Mild acute illness or antibiotic use is not a contraindication to immunization. MMR is not contraindicated in children of pregnant women. OPV, but not MMR, is contraindicated in any household contact of a severely immunocompromised person. In fact, in an effort to reduce vaccine-associated paralytic polio (VAPP), OPV is no longer recommended for the first two doses of polio immunizations in infants since 1997, and effective January 2000, the CDC recommendations are to give 4 doses of IPV at 2 months, 4 months, 6–18 months, and then at 6–8 years. OPV can be considered only under a few specific circumstances. If the parents refuse the schedule, OPV could be given only for the third or fourth dose and parents should be counseled about the possible occurrence of VAPP. In this case scenario, however, OPV would not be acceptable given the sibling situation. Live and inactivated vaccines can be given at the same time.

135. The answer is a. *(Chin, 17/e, pp 76–78. Fauci, 14/e, p 970.)* Prevention of human brucellosis depends on pasteurization of dairy products from cows, goats, and sheep; education of farmers and workers in the livestock industry as to the dangers of infected animals; and care in handling products from aborted animals. There is no insect vector. No vaccine for human use is available. Since person-to-person transmission does not occur, treatment of individual cases will not control spread of brucellosis. Destruction of infected animals will prevent transmission to other animals and is a method to control an outbreak in animals. Vaccine is available for livestock, for prevention but not control of outbreak. Vaccines have been used for workers in the meat and dairy industries in the former Soviet Union and Europe, but it is not used in the United States. Immunity from the vaccine lasts only two years.

136. The answer is b. *(CDC, Guidelines for Vaccinating Pregnant Women, 1998. Chin 17/e, pp 92, 96).* Varicella-zoster vaccine is a live attenuated vaccine. In general, live attenuated vaccines, such as the MMR, should be avoided during pregnancy because of the potential of infecting the fetus, which may result in congenital malformation. If a susceptible pregnant woman comes in contact with varicella, the administration of varicella-zoster immunoglobulin (VZIG) should be strongly considered because the disease can be very severe for women during pregnancy. However, there is no assurance that VZIG may prevent congenital infection and malformation, a relatively rare event (risk 0.7% if acquired early in pregnancy and 2% if acquired between 12 and 20 weeks of gestation). Because neonates are at risk of developing severe generalized varicella, VZIG is also indicated for newborns of mothers who develop chicken pox 5 days prior to or within 48 hours after delivery. Hepatitis B and influenza vaccines are inactivated and should be administered to women at risk of infection. Both vaccines available for the prophylaxis of rabies are inactivated and should be given to pregnant women when indicated. Tetanus toxoid and diphtheria toxoid are the only immunobiological agents routinely indicated for susceptible pregnant women. Previously vaccinated pregnant women who have not received a Td vaccination within the last 10 years should receive a booster dose.

137. The answer is e. *(CDC, MMWR 40[RR-12], 1991.)* If a person has received three doses or more of the Td, and the last dose was given more than five years before an injury, a tetanus and diphtheria booster should be given if the wound is contaminated, such as the one described. It is preferable to administer the combined diphtheria and tetanus booster (Td). You are then also using the opportunity to provide primary prevention for diphtheria. If the last dose of Td was given in the preceding five years, then no further action would be necessary. Td and tetanus immunoglobulin

(TIG) are recommended for prophylaxis of contaminated wounds when the history of tetanus toxoid is unknown or the person received less than three doses. TIG is never recommended as sole prophylaxis as prolonged immunity is desired.

138. The answer is d. (*Chin, 17/e, pp 374, 543.*) The infectious agent for epidemic forms of typhus fever is *Rickettsia prowazekii*, which is transmitted from person to person by the human body louse, *Pediculus humanus corporis*. Disruptions of social and economic institutions by war, famine, or natural catastrophes are associated with declining standards of personal hygiene and spread of lice. Even before social and economic recovery after World War II, epidemic typhus was controlled by mass application of DDT powder. This insecticide killed the body lice; thus, the transmission cycle was interrupted. Widespread resistance to DDT and lindane now exists, and other products such as permethrin should be used. Effective antibiotic therapy with chloramphenicol and tetracycline was not available until the early 1950s. *Anopheles* mosquitoes are vectors in the transmission of malaria, not typhus.

139. The answer is c. (*Chin, 17/e, pp 166–168.*) Diphtheria toxoid, alone or in combination with pertussis vaccine and tetanus toxoid (DTaP), induces protective levels of antitoxin that persist for about 10 years. Boosters are required every 10 years after completion of primary immunization in order to maintain protective concentration of antibody. Antitoxin antibodies do not prevent infection of the respiratory tract with *C. diphtheriae* and do not prevent the development of the carrier state. The antibodies are directed against the exotoxin produced by the bacteria, not against the bacteria themselves. Adverse reactions from the toxoid are very infrequent in infants and young children but are more common in adults; therefore, the administration of a reduced dose of toxoid is recommended for children after their seventh birthday and for adults. The reduced dose is symbolized by a lowercase *d.* It is usually combined with tetanus toxoid as a Td.

140. The answer is d. (*CDC, MMWR 47[RR-8], 1998.*) What's important here is to remember the concept that passively acquired measles antibody can interfere with the immune response of the measles vaccine. The intervals suggested by CDC are extrapolated from an estimated half-life of 30 days for passively acquired antibody and an observed interference with the immune response to measles vaccine for five months after a dose of 80 mg IgG/kg. The intervals vary according to the amount of plasma (containing the antibodies) or immunoglobulins present in the preparations. The recommended interval is 0 months for washed red cell transfusion; 3 months for adenine-saline RBC transfusion; 6 months for packed RBCs or whole blood; and 7 months for plasma/platelet transfusion. An interval of 3 months is recommended between the administration of tetanus immunoglobulin (TIG), hepatitis A prophylaxis with serum immunoglobulin (IG), and hepatitis B immunoglobulin (HBIG), and the MMR vaccine; 4 months between human rabies immunoglobulin (HRIG) and the MMR vaccine; and 5 months between varicella zoster immunoglobulin (VZIG) and MMR.

141. The answer is e. *(Holmes, 3/e, pp 1117–1120. Eur. Mod. Deliv. Collab. Lancet 353, 1999.)* The landmark randomized placebo controlled trial ACTG 076 demonstrated that zidovudine (ZDV) given at the beginning of the second trimester, during labor and delivery, and to the newborn for 6 weeks, significantly reduced the transmission of HIV to the newborn from 25.5% in the control group to 8.3% in the treatment group. Thus, ZDV can be highly effective for primary prevention in the newborn. Other promising treatment schedules with ZDV and other antiretrovirals are under study. Recent data demonstrates that a cesarean section can reduce vertical transmission, but it should not supersede antiretroviral therapy. Currently, it appears that it is not a routinely recommended procedure for HIV-infected pregnant women, but this may change in the future. HIV can be transmitted by breast feeding, and in some studies, the risk is increased by 14%. However, breast feeding has no impact on the highest risk of transmission, which occurs during gestation, labor, and delivery. Early identification of newborns at risk of HIV infection will guide the medical management and improve outcomes. It has no impact on the primary prevention of the infection to the newborn. Finally, all HIV-infected women should be made aware of the benefit of ZDV so they can make informed choices.

142. The answer is d. *(CDC, MMWR 48[RR-7], 1999.)* Nantucket Island (off the coast of Massachusetts) has one of the highest rates of Lyme disease in the United States. Lyme disease is a tick-borne zoonosis from the spirochete *Borelia burgdorferi*. Avoidance of bushy areas is the first line of prevention recommendation for patients traveling in endemic areas. Risk is higher in summer and spring. However, it is unrealistic to expect this patient to keep away from bushy areas. His best protection would be wearing appropriate clothing and applying DEET to avoid tick bites. Next, since infection rarely occurs if the tick has been attached for less than 36 hours, daily checks for ticks may be helpful. Antibiotics are used for treatment but not prophylaxis. Optimal protection for the vaccine is obtained after three doses at 0, 1, and 12 months. Vaccine is currently primarily recommended for persons 15 to 70 who engage in activities that result in *prolonged* exposure to tick-infested habitat in areas of high to moderate risk. Benefit of the vaccine for short exposure beyond that provided by personal protection is uncertain. Furthermore, there would not be enough time to complete the series in this case.

143–144. The answers are 143-b, 144-d. *(Holmes, 3/e, pp 1081.)* *Chlamydia trachomatis* is the most frequently reported bacterial sexually transmitted disease (STD) in the United States. Infections of the cervix may present as a friable cervix, but are most often without signs or symptoms. Pelvic inflammatory disease (PID) caused by chlamydia often presents with milder symptoms than when it is caused by gonorrhea. Prompt treatment reduces the occurrence of long-term sequelae such as infertility, ectopic pregnancy, and chronic pelvic pain. The risk of infertility appears to be higher for chlamydial infections compared to any other STD. Screening women is important to reduce the risk of PID and its sequelae.

145. The answer is e. *(Holmes, 3/e, p 368. Fauci [full text], 14/e, pp 1679–1681.)* Currently available laboratory tests for hepatitis B include HBsAg (hepatitis B surface antigen), anti-HBs (antibody to hepatitis B surface antigen), IgM anti-HBc, IgG anti-HBc (antibodies to the core antigen), HBeAg, and anti-HBe. Because HBcAg is sequestered within an HBsAg coat, HBcAg is not routinely detected in patients with hepatitis B. IgM anti-HBc appears soon after the onset of infection and the detection of HBsAg, and precedes by many weeks detectable levels of anti-HBsAg. It generally disappears after 6 to 8 months. The presence of IgM is a marker for acute (less than 6 months) hepatitis B. IgG anti-HBc appears somewhat later than the IgM and may persist for years. Elevated ALT may be present both in the early and chronic phases of the disease. HBeAg may persist for years in patients with chronic disease and is associated with high infectivity. HBsAg remains detectable beyond 6 months in chronic hepatitis B.

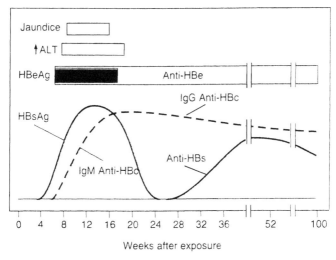

A

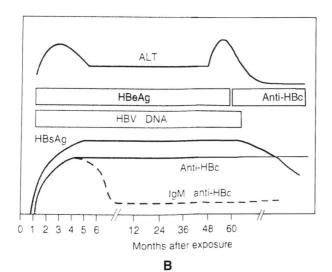

B

(Reproduced, with permission, from Dienstag JL, Isselbacher KJ. Acute viral hepatitis. In: Fauci AS, Braunwald E, Isselbacher KJ, eds., *Harrison's Principles of Internal Medicine,* 14th ed., New York, McGraw-Hill, 1998: 1680.)

146–148. The answers are 146-c, 147-a, 148-d. *(Fauci, 14/e [companion book], pp 447–449. CDC, MMWR 49[RR-8]: 149–153, 2000.)* The incidence of nosocomial infections in acute care hospitals is estimated to be 3 to 5% of patients admitted, costing the system close to $2 billion per year. The most frequent adult site is the urinary tract, followed by ventilator-associated pneumonia, surgical wounds, and septicemia. The single most important risk factor is hand washing. Restricting invasive procedures only to those who absolutely need it (such as catheterization) will reduce infections. Disinfection of sheets and towels already occurs in hospitals. Some specific ventilation requirements exist for acid-fast bacillus isolation (TB). Isolation is also necessary for certain conditions: strict isolation for varicella, contact isolation for staph wounds, respiratory isolation for untreated meningitis, and enteric precautions for infectious diarrhea, such as *C. difficile.*

149. The answer is d. *(Wallace, 14/e, p 214.)* In 1995, the proportion of active TB cases comprised of the foreign-born was 36% and this proportion has now risen. Conversion from latent to active disease among the foreign-born is 100 to 200 times that of the U.S. rate. TB is more prevalent in correctional settings (up to 25% of inmates have positive PPDs), among injecting drug users, and in the homeless population. HIV is a risk factor for TB.

150. The answer is a. *(Holmes, 3/e, p 368. Chin, 17/e, p 244.)* The likelihood of becoming chronically infected with hepatitis B is inversely related to the age at which the infection occurs. Up to 90% of infants born to HBsAg-positive mothers will become carriers. Between 25 and 50% of children infected before the age of 5 will become carriers. Only 6 to 10% of acutely infected adults become chronically infected. The risk of becoming a chronic carrier is the same for men and women. Parenteral transmission is not associated with a higher risk of chronic disease compared with sexual transmission. Although antigen dose may affect the risk of acquiring hepatitis B, it has no impact on chronic carrier status. Immunodeficiency can affect response to vaccine and can be a risk factor for chronic carrier status following an acute infection, but not to the same degree as young age.

151–153. The answers are 151-b, 152-e, 153-e. *(Chin, 17/e, pp 340–345. CDC, MMWR 46[RR-5]: 1–21, 1997.)* The case fatality rate for meningococcemia has decreased dramatically with prompt antibiotic therapy and supportive measures. Meningococcemia and meningococcal meningitis are both reportable diseases and carry the same risk of transmission. The risk of developing disease is much higher among household contacts than in the general population. For sporadic cases, prompt administration of appropriate antibiotic prophylaxis is recommended for household contacts; those in contact with oral secretions, such as those sharing utensils or kissing; close friends at school (but not all classmates); and *all* day care contacts, both adults and children. Rifampin is the agent of choice for adults and children. Other choices include ceftriaxone for adults and children. Ciprofloxacin can be given only to nonpregnant adults. Antibiotics should be administered promptly, ideally within 24 hours of case identification. Vaccination would not be an acceptable option for this case since it takes too long to develop antibodies and protection. It is used to control outbreaks in large settings, communities, and colleges. The serogroup C component of the vaccine is poorly immunogenic in children under the age of 2.

154–155. The answer is 154-a, 155-d. *(Holmes, 3/e, p 479. CDC, MMWR 47[RR-1] 1998.)* Nontreponemal tests RPR, VDRL can be negative in up to 30% of patients at an initial visit for primary syphilis. The probability of a negative test is increased if the patient presents early in the course of primary syphilis. The FTA-ABS, a treponemal test, is more sensitive and is reactive around the time of appearance of the lesion. The dark-field is the investigation of first choice to confirm a diagnosis of syphilis when a chancre is present. Both nontreponemal and treponemal tests will become reactive within three weeks after the chancre has occurred. The incubation period for syphilis is between 10 and 90 days, with an average of 21 days. The lesion typical of chancroid is a large and painful ulcer with undermined borders. Large inguinal adenopathy, often suppurative, is also present. The incubation period is usually between 4 and 7 days. Herpetic lesions are shallow, painful, and multiple. Donovanosis is very rare in developed countries and is characterized by lesions that slowly enlarge, bleed easily on contact, and often have beefy-red granulomatous tissue. Lymphogranuloma venereum is also uncommon. It is primarily a disease of the lymphatic system. Patients often present with complaints related to inguinal adenopathy. The initial lesion, which is small, shallow, and painless, often goes unnoticed. For primary syphilis, sexual partners from the previous three months since the onset of symptoms should be assessed (6 months for secondary syphilis, and 12 months for early latent).

156. The answer is c. *(Fauci, 14/e [companion book], p 566.)* Erythema infectiosum (EI), caused by parvovirus type B19, is a mild, limited viral infection characterized by a distinctive rash on the face often called "slapped-cheek" because of its intensity. The infection may cause chronic anemia in immunodeficient persons and aplastic crisis in those with chronic hemolytic anemia. Adenoviruses cause upper respiratory tract infections and occasionally severe pneumonia. Adenovirus types 31, 40, and 41 have been associated with gastroenteritis. Coxsackieviruses cause multiple clinical manifestations. Type A16 causes the hand, foot, and mouth syndrome, and type A24 has been associated with hemorrhagic conjunctivitis. Rotaviruses are implicated in diarrheal syndromes, and echovirus 9 in petechial exanthem and meningitis. Coxsackieviruses and echoviruses are nonpolio enteroviruses.

157. The answer is a. *(CDC, MMWR 47[RR-8], 1998.)* Unusual or serious adverse events following the administration of the MMR have not been documented in HIV-infected children who were not severely immunocompromised. Because measles may cause a severe infection in HIV-infected persons, vaccination is recommended if no immunosupression is present. Live vaccines should be avoided during pregnancy. Patients with leukemia in remission may receive live vaccines only if chemotherapy has been terminated for at least three months. An oral dose of 2 mg/kg or 20 mg of prednisone for two weeks or more is considered sufficient to induce immunosuppression and warrants concern about the safety of administration of a live vaccine.

158–159. The answers are 158-a, 159-d. *(CDC, MMWR 40[RR-50]: 929–933, 1995.)* Overall, the risk of HIV transmission following a percutaneous injury is 0.3%. A case-control study conducted with cases from the United States, France, and the United Kingdom demonstrated that the factor associated with the greatest risk of transmission of HIV to the health care worker following a needle-stick injury was the depth of the injury (odds ratio 16.1, confidence interval 6.1–44.6). In addition, the presence of blood on the device, terminal illness in the source patient, and a procedure that required placing the needle directly in a vein or artery were also associated with a higher risk of transmission. Postexposure use of zidovudine decreased the risk of transmission. Guidelines on prophylaxis following a percutaneous injury have been issued by the CDC (*MMWR 1998; 47[RR-7]: 1–28*) and include triple therapy.

160. The answer is c. *(Chin, 17/e, pp 375–378.)* Pertussis has been recognized with increased frequency in the United States among young adults and adolescents who were previously immunized. The immunity provided by the vaccine is limited and fades over time. The infection can be particularly severe in children under the age of 1. Antibiotic prophylaxis with erythromycin is recommended for all household and close contacts to prevent disease and outbreaks. The symptoms are not typical of influenza, legionellosis, or pneumonia due to streptococci. Prophylaxis of contacts is not recommended for mycoplasma infections; it is much less contagious than pertussis.

161. The answer is d. *(Chin, 17/e, p 39. CDC, MMWR 48[39]: 871–874, 1999.)* All the others causes of meningitis are viral and arthropod-borne (mosquitoes). An outbreak of the recently described Nile-like encephalitis occurred in New York City starting in August of 1999 and required application of mosquito control compounds.

162. The answer is e. *(Chin, 17/e, p 340.)* With widespread use of the vaccine, *Haemophilus meningitis*, once the leading cause of bacterial meningitis in children, has practically been eliminated in the United States. The most common cause in now *N. meningitidis* followed by *S. pneumoniae*. Meningitis caused by other etiologic agents occurs in susceptible individuals such as neonates and immunosuppressed persons, or is the result of head trauma.

163. The answer is c. *(Chin, 17/e, pp 238–257.)* Hepatitis C is primarily parenterally transmitted and a high percentage of intravenous drug users are found to be infected. Hepatitis A and E are transmitted via the fecal/oral route and result in similar self-limited acute symptomatic episodes. Hepatitis E is rare in the United States, occurring among travellers returning from endemic countries such Asia, India, Africa, and Central America. Living conditions of intravenous drug users may also increase the risk of them acquiring such infections, but hepatitis C is much more prevalent. Hepatitis D only occurs with coinfection with hepatitis B. The presence of antibody against hepatitis B signals a past infection and clearance of the virus.

164. The answer is b. *(Chin, 17/e, pp 270–272. Greenberg, 2/e, p 70.)* Antigenic drift is most likely the cause of changes in the strain that allowed infection despite adequate vaccination. Partial immunity or mutation to a less-virulent strain (also due to antigenic drift) could be responsible for the less severe symptoms noted in this outbreak. Antigenic drift is a slow and progressive change in the antigenic composition of microorganisms. This alters the immunological responses of individuals and a population's susceptibility to that microorganism. Antigenic shift is a sudden change in the molecular structure of a microorganism and produces new strains. This results in little or no acquired immunity to these new strains and is the explanation for new epidemics or pandemics. Vaccine failure would result in influenza cases with high case fatality rates seen previously with this strain. Herd immunity would decrease the rate of infection by decreasing the probability that a susceptible person would come into contact with an infected person. This would not affect the clinical presentation of those infected. Influenza is not a rhinovirus and there is no cross-immunity between the two.

165. The answer is e. *(Fauci, 14/e [full text], pp 1826–1827. CDC, MMWR 47[RR-20], 1998.)* The management of HIV infection is a rapidly evolving field as new scientific information emerges and new drugs are developed. As of 1999, prophylaxis for *P. carinii* remains the recommendation for patients with a CD4 + T cell count of under 200/μL or CD4 % of less than 15%. Prophylaxis for MAC should begin when the CD4 cell count is less than 100/μL or 50μL. Prophylaxis for cryptococcus is optional depending on the risk and should be given when CD4 counts are less than 50/μL. Because the medications used for toxoplasmosis have severe side effects, they do not make good choices for primary prophylaxis. Fortunately, patients receiving trimethoprim/sulfamethoxazole or dapsone or pyrimethamine for prophylaxis of PCP have a decreased incidence of toxoplasmosis. Candidates for TB preventive therapy in HIV-infected persons include persons with a PPD ≥5 mm who have not previously received treatment for TB, persons with a contact with an infectious case, persons with prior untreated/inadequately treated/healed without treatment TB, and persons at high risk of acquiring TB because of living in jails or homeless shelters.

166. The answer is d. *(Greenberg, 2/e, pp 63–69.)* The identification of a specific factor (food) as a cause of illness (food poisoning) depends on comparing the proportion who become ill among those who did and those who did not eat each specified food (the proportion ill is sometimes called the "attack rate," but in fact it is a proportion, not a rate). The proportion ill among those who ate the food suspected of causing the disease should be significantly greater than among those who did not eat the food.

167. The answer is a. *(Chin, 17/e, p 3. Fauci [full text], 14/e, pp 1798, 1800.)* In the United States, men who have sex with men still account for the largest proportion of cumulative cases. However, the epidemic has been shifting since the mid-1990s, as women and minorities accounted for the largest increase in newly reported rates. Despite advances in treatment, resulting in an overall decrease in HIV-related deaths in the United States, AIDS remains the leading cause of death for all men and women between the ages of 25 and 44.

168. The answer is d. *(Chin, 17/e, p 218. CDC JAMA 282: 2113–2114, 1999.)* The rotavirus vaccine was rapidly removed from the market (a few months after the CDC had recommended its use) because of reports of intussusception ocurring in infants within three weeks of vaccination.

169. The answer is b. *(Chin, 17/e, pp 567, 572.)* The incubation period is the duration of time between exposure to an infectious agent and the appearance of the first manifestation of the disease. In contrast, the decubation period is the time from the disappearance of symptoms until recovery and the absence of infectious organisms. The communicable period designates the time when the infected person can transmit the infectious agent to another person.

170. The answer is e. *(Chin, 17/e, pp 155–157.)* The symptoms described are consistent with an infection with the enterohemorrhagic strain *E. coli* H157:H7, complicated by thrombotic thrombocytopenic purpura (TTP). It can also be complicated by the hemolytic uremic syndrome (HUS) in 2 to 7% of cases. It occurs mostly in children. Outbreaks most often have been associated with consumption of inadequately cooked hamburger from fast-food restaurants. Raw milk contaminated by cattle feces or unpasteurized apple cider can also be sources. Cattle are the reservoir. The lack of fever helps differentiate this from shigellosis and dysenteria caused by other strains of *E. coli* or *Campylobacter.*

171–173. The answers are 171-d, 172-a, 173-b. *(CDC, MMWR 47[RR-19]: 1–39, 1998.)* CDC recommends routine screening for persons who have ever used injecting drugs, who have received transfusions or organ transplants before July 1992, who received clotting factor concentrates prior to 1987, who were ever on long-term dialysis, and who have persistently abnormal alanine aminotransferase I (ALT) levels. Health care and emergency personnel should be routinely tested only if exposed. If the screening EIA is positive, a confirmation assay with an immunoblot should be performed. If this is also positive, it should be followed by qualitative and quantitative HCV RNA determination to guide evaluation for treatment. No prohylaxis is available for newborns of infected mothers. Co-infection with HIV increases the risk of vertical transmission to 15%. Mode of delivery does not appear to affect transmission rates. Passively transferred antibodies to HCV can remain in the offspring for up to 12 months; therefore, the EIA should not be used for diagnosis during that time. No transmission by breast milk has been documented.

174–175. The answers are 174-d, 175-e. (*CDC, MMWR 48[RR-12]: 1–37, 1999.*) RNA quantification is not generally used for diagnostic purposes, but rather for typing strains and epidemiologic research. IgM antibodies can be detected 5 to 10 days *before* the onset of symptoms and must be present to confirm a diagnosis of hepatitis A. They persist for 6 months. Commercial tests are also available for the detection of total antibodies (IgG and IgM). IgG antibodies are detectable early in disease, persist for life, and provide lifelong immunity. Children, because they are often asymptomatic of the disease, play an important role in the transmission of the infection. In one study of adults for whom no source of infection was identified, 52% had children under age six and the presence of a young child in the household was associated with HAV transmission. In this situation, children should be tested as well as other household contacts. Most cases of hepatitis A in the United States result from person-to-person transmission: 11 to 26% from either household or sexual contact, and 11 to 16% from day care settings. An additional 4 to 6% are reported from international travelers, and 2 to 3% from recognized water- or foodborne disease outbreaks. Outbreaks have also occurred among injecting drug users and men who have sex with men.

176. The answer is b. (*Chin, 17/e, p 442. Fauci, 14/e [companion volume], pp 402–403.*) Persons with sickle cell disease have functional asplenism due to infarction. This results in impaired immune response to polysaccharide antigens, such as *Streptococcus pneumoniae, H. influenza,* and *N. meningitidis.* They are more susceptible to invasive *Salmonella* infection, which is often not preceded by enteric symptoms. Localization of a systemic infection often results in osteomyelitis. Persons with sickle cell disease are also more susceptible to malaria.

177. The answer is b. *(Holmes, 3/e, pp 285–289.)* In fact, over 80% of persons who are HSV-2 seropositve do not know that they are infected. Many of these have atypical symptoms and signs while some are completely asymptomatic. Up to 30% of genital infections in the United States are caused by HSV type 1, which does not recur as often as type 2. Most transmissions occur when patients are asymptomatic. Shedding between clinical episodes is common and is more likely to occur in the first year after the acquisition of the infection. The presence of genital ulcers can increase the risk of acquiring and transmitting HIV. Type-specific serology tests are now commercially available (POCkit® and Meridian®).

178. The answer is e. *(CDC, MMWR 48[RR-1]: 5–7, 1999.)* Two doses of vaccine IM, one immediately and one 3 days later, are recommended for those who were previously immunized. A primary course of vaccination consists of three doses of one of the three approved vaccines at 0, 7, and 21 or 28 days. It is recommended for persons in high-risk groups such as veterinarians, animal handlers, and certain laboratory personnel.

179–180. The answers are 179-a, 180-e. *(Chin, 17/e, pp 92–97. CDC, MMWR 48[RR-6]: 2, 1999.)* The most common serious complication of varicella is pneumonia, followed by encephalitis. Thrombocytopenia has been associated mainly with rubella. Reye's syndrome was a frequent complication to varicella before the association with aspirin was discovered. Varicella-zoster immune globulin is recommended for susceptible pregnant women as the infection may be more severe during pregnancy. It is not clear whether it can prevent congenital infection if exposure occurred earlier in pregnancy. It must be given within 96 hours of exposure. Furthermore, infection may be very severe in newborns of mothers who develop the infection either 5 days prior to or within 48 hours after delivery. Given the mean incubation period of 14 to 16 days, the mother may develop the infection just at the time of delivery if no prophylaxis is given. VZIG would also be indicated for the sibling. Vaccine has been shown effective in controlling outbreaks which otherwise can last for months. The Advisory Committee on Immunization Practices (ACIP) now recommends that states require children to either have received vaccine or have evidence of immunity from varicella before entering child care facilities or elementary school. Varicella vaccine is a live attenuated vaccine and is contraindicated during pregnancy.

181. The answer is b. *(Holmes, 3/e, p 1174.)* The clinical picture of "snuffles," a persistent often sanguinous nasal discharge, is associated with congenital syphilis in addition to hepatosplenomegaly, anemia, and anomalies of the long bones visible by x-ray. Congenital rubella is associated with deafness, cataracts, microcephaly, and heart defects. Chorioretinitis and brain damage with intracerebral calcifications are seen in toxoplasmosis and CMV infections. Congenital varicella is extremely uncommon.

182. The answer is a. *(CDC, MMWR 48[RR-4]: 15–18, 1999.)* Amantadine and rimantadine are indicated for the prevention and treatment of influenza A only. They are 70 to 90% effective in preventing disease, though they are not substitutes for vaccination. When an outbreak occurs in a nursing home, all residents should receive chemoprophylaxis, regardless of vaccination status. They could still be vaccinated, but antibodies are produced only after two weeks. Unvaccinated staff should also be offered chemoprophylaxis. If a variant strain is suspected that is not well matched with the vaccine, then all staff should be offered prophylaxis.

183. The answer is a. *(AAP, 2000.)* Pneumococcal vaccine PPV23 is not effective in children less than 2 years of age. A heptavalent pneumococcal conjugate vaccine (PCV7) has been approved for use in children 23 months and younger. PCV7 is now recommended for universal use for all children under 23 months, including those at high risk (which includes HIV infection). Other indications for pneumococcal vaccine include persons over the age of 65 and those with anatomical or functional asplenia, nephrotic syndrome, sickle cell disease, chronic heart and lung disease, cirrhosis of the liver, and diabetes. As this is a rapidly evolving field and includes more complicated regimens for children, consultation with local health departments should be made for the latest recommendations for immunization series and boosters.

184. The answer is c. *(MDPH 1999.)* Common-source, also known as point-source (for example, guests at a wedding reception), outbreaks typically give an epidemic curve with a sharp rise followed by a decline usually less abrupt. The epidemic curve from a propagated-source or person-to-person outbreak (for example, community outbreak of shigellosis) is characterized by rather slow progressive rise. The curve will continue for several incubation periods of the disease. The continual-source outbreak (for example, food continuously contaminated by food handlers) is characterized by continual peaks over time. Peaks are not as dramatic as for common-source, and the outbreak may not be as obvious.

185. The answer is b. *(Chin, 17/e, pp 215–218.)* Rotavirus is the most common cause of gastroenteritis as well as dehydration in children. Peak occurrence is between 6 and 24 months. The diarrhea is more severe than that caused by other organisms. In temperate climates, rotavirus infections peak during cooler months (sporadic and seasonal).

186. The answer is b. *(CDC, MMWR 47[RR-20]: 18–22, 1998. Chin, 17/e, pp 526–527.)* HIV-infected persons are at high risk of tuberculosis and should be screened on a regular basis. An induration of 5 mm or more on a skin test is considered positive if the patient is HIV-infected, has had contact with an infectious TB disease case, or has an abnormal chest x-ray suggesting old, healed TB. The patient in this example is asymptomatic and the chest x-ray is normal, suggesting latent infection as opposed to active disease. Prophylaxis is warranted. Long-course preventive treatment (9 to 12 months) with izoniazid (INH) is recommended for HIV-infected persons. Short-course preventive therapy (2 months) with rifampin and pyrazinamide or izoniazid has also been shown to be effective. However, rifampin can significantly reduce circulating blood levels of protease inhibitors and is therefore contraindicated in patients taking these antiretrovirals.

187. The answer is a. *(CDC, MMWR 47[RR-20]: 4–5, 1998.)* Overlap between the AIDS and TB epidemics continues to contribute to the increase in TB morbidity. HIV seropositivity is a risk factor for resistance to all first-line drugs for TB, particularly INH, rifampin, or both drugs. The reason is that recently acquired TB, which is more likely to be drug-resistant, is more common with HIV-infected persons than reactivated TB. Up to 11% of HIV-infected persons may have resistance to INH, about 9% to rifampin, and 6% to both.

188. The answer is a. (*CDC, MMWR 47[RR-20]: 28–29, 1998.*) Directly observed (health care worker supervises and observes intake of medication) initial-phase therapy with a four drug regimen of izoniazid, rifampin, ethambutol, and pyrazinamide is recommended always. For patients on protease inhibitors or nonnucleoside reverse transcriptase inhibitors (NNRTI) therapy, rifampin should be substituted by rifambutin (shown to have little effect on circulating blood levels of these antiviral therapies). For those in whom rifamycins are contraindicated, the use of streptomycin as a substitute is recommended.

189. The answer is e. (*CDC, MMWR 48[RR-12], 1999.*) The effectiveness of the vaccine in controlling outbreaks in day care settings remains to be proven. Only if the center has children in diapers do all children and staff need immunoglobulin. Vaccine has been shown to be helpful in decreasing the number of expected cases of hepatitis A during large community outbreaks in areas where the prevalence of disease is high or moderate. Recommendations from CDC for routine vaccination will depend on the regional epidemiology of disease. The national average rate is 10 cases per 100,000 population. Areas with rates exceeding 20/100,000 include Alaska, New Mexico, Arizona, Oregon, Utah, and Washington, and are concentrated on the West Coast. Rates are particularly high among American Indian and Alaskan natives. CDC recommends that children living in states, communities, or counties where the rates are twice the national average be routinely vaccinated.

190. The answer is d. (*CDC, MMWR 47[RR-1] 1998.*) The rapid RPR card test can be done stat in the clinic. It is a qualitative test and will not provide titration information. However, given that the test is positive, there is no reason to further delay treatment of this patient (given her history and noncompliance in prenatal visits) while waiting to receive titers and treponemal test results. Penicillin is the *only* recommended treatment for syphilis during pregnancy and should be given a least four weeks before delivery to be effective in treating the fetus. Regimens are the same as for nonpregnant women. In this case, it would be prudent to treat as a case of late latent syphilis (no symptoms consistent with secondary or primary syphilis, and unable to confirm if early, that is, less than one-year duration). Women who are allergic should be desensitized under observation and treated with penicillin. A Jarisch-Xerheimer reaction can occur when treating early syphilis. This may precipitate contractions after the second trimester, so women should be observed. Erythromycin has an unacceptable cure rate and is no longer recommended. Doxycycline is contraindicated during pregnancy. Adequate regimens of ceftriaxone have not been defined.

191–192. The answers are 191-d, 192-c. *(Chin, 17/e, pp 134–137.)* People with normal immune function generally have asymptomatic or self-limited infections. AIDS patients may be unable to clear the infection which can then have a prolonged and fulminant course. Chemical disinfection is ineffective against oocysts and only filters removing particles of 0.1 to 1 microns will eliminate *C. parvum*. Boiling water for 1 minute is effective, inexpensive, and easy to achieve. The quality of bottled water may be unreliable and is not a practical public health approach.

193. The answer is e. *(Holmes, 3/e, p 407.)* Women are particularly at risk of developing complications for the disease and should be the first group to be targeted for screening. Age has consistently been shown to be a risk factor for disease, regardless of the other behaviors described. Women under the age of 20 should be screened at *any* pelvic examination, and at least once a year. Some experts recommend screening every six months. Sexually active women between the ages of 20 and 24 should be screened every year, again regardless of presence or absence of risky behaviors. Since most chlamydial infections are asymptomatic in both men and women, most transmissions occur among persons who are unknowingly infected. The Health Employment Data and Information Set (HEDIS), which measures quality among HMOs, now has a chlamydia screening quality indicator: the proportion of sexually active women between the ages of 15 and 24 who are screened annually for *C. trachomatis.* When symptoms are present, the test is diagnostic. Screening, by definition, is the detection of a condition before symptoms occur.

194. The answer is d. *(Holmes, 3/e, pp 454, 459–460.)* The gram stain shows more than 4 PMNs per high power field (one of the diagnostic criteria for urethritis) as well as the presence of gram negative *intracellular* (extracellular are less specific) diplococci (GNID), which is diagnostic for the presence of *Neisseria gonorrhoeae.* The gram stain is 90 to 95% sensitive and 95 to 100% specific for the detection of gonorrhea in men presenting with urethritis. Cultures should be done to confirm diagnosis and assess antibiotic susceptibility. The test performance characteristics of the gram stain to detect gonorrhea in the cervix of women are not as good (only 50 to 70% sensitive). Therefore, the absence of GNID on a cervical sample does not rule out gonorrhea. The incubation period for gonorrhea is 1 to 14 days, with an average of 2 to 5 days. This patient should be given a regimen recommended for gonorrhea (ceftriaxone, cefixime, or a quinolone) as well as one for chlamydia because coinfections can be as high as 40% in certain settings.

195. The answer is d. (*Chin, 17/e, pp 75–77, 521–525.*) Clinical symptoms caused by *M. bovis* are indistinguishable from those of *M. tuberculosis*. This patient is unlikely to have been in contact with someone with active TB, given that he lives in rural areas. His occupation, however, may lead to contact with *M. bovis*. Brucellosis may also cause fever, sweats, fatigue, but is not associated with cough. The incubation period generally does not exceed two months.

196. The answer is c. (*Chin, 17/e, pp 248, 346, 377, 402.*) Immunization schedules recommended by the CDC have evolved rapidly in the last two years and are becoming increasingly complicated. The state health department should keep providers up to date. As of early 2000, the schedule described in C is recommended for children born to HBsAG-positive mothers. These children should receive HBIG and the first dose of vaccine within 12 hours of birth, the second dose of vaccine at 1–2 months of age, and the third dose at 6 months of age. Schedules may differ for mothers who are HBsAG-negative (see answers to questions 231–232). OPV is no longer recommended (see question 134). Acellular preparations (DTaP) that contain two or more protective antigens of *B. pertussis* are used in the United States for primary series and boosters.

197. The answer is d. (*Holmes, 3/e, pp 450–356.*) Recurrence of infection is primarily associated with host factors, and studies have shown that treating male partners of females with human papillomavirus (HPV) infections will have no impact on the recurrence of disease. Recurrence rates are higher in the first year (about 30%) and decline afterward (9% in the second year). Unfortunately, there is no convincing data that condoms effectively prevent infection, although these studies are difficult to conduct. Part of the issue is that the condom may not cover all areas infected with the virus. However, condom use should continue to be encouraged for the prevention of other STDs and HIV (where they have been shown to be effective). There is no data to suggest that treating external genital warts will reduce the risk of cervical cancer. In fact, most external lesions are caused by nononcogenic types of HPV such as type 6 or 11. This patient should not be screened more frequently than women without external warts if her Pap smears are normal. She should be encouraged to be screened on a yearly basis.

198–200.   The answers are 198-b, 199-d, 200-a. (*Chin, 17/e, pp 412, 405–406, 441–442, 272, 524, 331, 137, 559, 79.*) Rabies, psittacosis, and salmonellosis are zoonoses, that is, infections transmitted from animals to humans. The reservoirs of rabies include domestic and wild canines, cats, skunks, raccoons, bats, and other biting mammals. Psittacosis is a zoonosis involving birds such as parakeets, parrots, pigeons, turkeys, and other domestic fowl. *Salmonella* species infect poultry, rodents, dogs, cats, and birds. (*S. typhi* is an exception in that no animal hosts are known.)

Tuberculosis, influenza, and measles are transmitted through airborne droplet spread. Only measles could also be spread by direct person-to-person contact.

Cyclospora, Campylobacter, and *Yersinia* have been implicated in waterborne outbreaks.

201–204.   The answers are 201-a, 202-b, 203-d, 204-c. (*Chin, 17/e, pp xxi–xxiii.*) *Immunogenicity* is a term that describes the ability of a microbe or purified antigen to induce specific antibody production in a host as a result of infection or immunization. For example, measles virus is very immunogenic because most persons develop neutralizing antibody, which persists for life following a single infection.

Pathogenicity is the capacity of a microbe to cause symptomatic illness in an infected host. The enormous numbers of nonpathogenic bacteria (up to 10^{10} per gram of colonic contents present in the human body) and the normal flora on the human body's external surface do not cause disease.

Virulence refers to the severity of illness produced by a microbe and is measured by the percentage of severe or fatal cases. Virulence may vary depending on the defenses of the host; for example, malnutrition impairs defenses against infection. In malnourished children, measles has a case-fatality rate of up to 10% compared with less than 0.1% in well-nourished children.

Infectivity (or *contagiousness*) of a microbe refers to the ability of a microbe to spread in a population of exposed susceptible persons. The secondary attack rate, that is, the incidence of a disease in contacts of a case, often is used to assess contagiousness.

205–207.   The answers are 205-a, 206-b, 207-c. *(CDC, STD surveillance report 1999.)* *Chlamydia trachomatis* is the most frequently reported bacterial STD in the United States. The number of reported cases has increased largely due to the increase in the number of states that have made chlamydia a reportable disease. With an emphasis on screening, rates may also increase in the coming years due to increased detection among asymptomatic persons. Gonococcal infections have been gradually decreasing since the mid-1980s, with a slight increase noted in the last two years. Syphilis has been decreasing since its peak in 1990, thought to be the result of increased drug use, particularly crack cocaine. It is not evenly distributed in the United States and is mainly concentrated in the southeast United States. The CDC has embarked on a syphilis elimination project in an effort to eradicate this infection within the next 10 years.

208–210.   The answers are 208-a, 209-c, 210-d. *(Chin, 17/e, pp 158– 160, 202–207.)* Staphylococcal food poisoning is caused by a heat-stable enterotoxin produced when staphylococci multiply in food. The incubation period is usually 2 to 4 h, and the illness is characterized by the sudden onset of severe nausea, vomiting, cramps, prostration, and diarrhea.

Most cases of traveler's diarrhea are caused by enterotoxin-producing strains of *Escherichia coli*. Although the mechanism of action of *E. coli* enterotoxin is similar to that of cholera enterotoxin, disease due to the former is usually not as severe. Disease due to *E. coli* enterotoxin is most common in regions of the world where adequate sanitation and pure water supplies are absent. Norfloxacin 400 mg daily has been shown to be effective in preventing disease. Alternatively, it may be preferable to initiate early treatment with the onset of diarrhea with either ciprofloxacin 500 mg BID or norfloxacin 400 mg daily for 5 days. These antibiotics are preferable for initiating treatment because many strains have been found to be resistant to other antimicrobials, such as sulfas or doxycycline.

Food poisoning caused by *Clostridium perfringens* usually has an incubation period of 10 to 12 h and is characterized by abrupt onset of abdominal colic followed by diarrhea. Vomiting is unusual, and the disease is usually of short duration. Outbreaks result from contamination of food during preparation and by improper cooking and storage; these circumstances allow bacteria to multiply which produce the enterotoxins. Food poisoning (or intoxication) caused by toxins elaborated by bacterial growth before consumption include *S. aureus, B. cereus,* and *C. botulinum.* Toxins causing the symptoms are produced by *C. perfringens* in the intestine once consumed.

211–213. The answers are 211-e, 212-d, 213-c. *(Chin, 17/e, pp 251, 253–254, 256.)* Hepatitis E is transmitted via the fecal/oral route. The clinical course of the disease is similar to that of hepatitis A, except in pregnant women, when the case fatality rate is high if the infection occurs in the third trimester. Cases in the United States are rare and have been documented only among travelers returning from countries where the illness is endemic. Hepatitis D can only replicate if coinfection with hepatitis B is present. Between 50 and 80% of adults who become infected with hepatitis C will develop chronic disease.

214–216. The answers are 214-c, 215-b, 216-e. *(Jekel, pp 35–40.)* *Endemic* refers to the constant presence or usual prevalence of a disease or infectious agent in a given geographic area. *Hyperendemic* refers to a constant presence of a very high incidence of disease/infection. *Epidemic* refers to the occurrence of disease/infection within a community clearly in excess of what is to be normally expected. A *pandemic* refers to widespread disease throughout a continent or across very large geographic areas or countries affecting very large numbers of people. *Zoonosis* refers to infection transmitted from other vertebrates to humans under natural conditions. They can be epizootic or endozootic (as in epidemic and endemic).

217–219. The answers are 217-d, 218-e, 219-b. *(Chin, 17/e, pp 370, 488, 497.)* Paragonimiasis is caused by the lung fluke, *Paragonimus westermani.* It has a complex life cycle in which larval stages undergo development in freshwater crabs and other crustacea. Infection occurs by eating infected raw crabs. The disease, which affects the lungs and causes chronic cough and hemoptysis, occurs primarily in the Far East but has recently been reported in the Western hemisphere.

Toxocariasis is caused by the dog roundworm, *Toxocara canis.* The disease occurs mainly in children as the result of ingestion of soil contaminated with *Toxocara* eggs. Development of *Toxocara* is incomplete in humans so that the larval stages migrate through the body—hence the term *visceral larva migrans.*

Cysticercosis is caused by the pork tapeworm, *Taenia solium.* Intestinal infection occurs by eating pork infested by cysts of *T. solium.* The adult tapeworm resides in the intestinal tract from which gravid proglottids (segments containing eggs) are shed in the feces. If the eggs hatch in the intestinal tract, the larvae can migrate throughout the body and often reach the brain. Cysticercosis is a common cause of epilepsy in Mexico and other developing countries.

220–224. The answers are 220-g, 221-c, 222-a, 223-b, 224-f. *(Chin, 17/e, pp 362, 232, 76, 187, 501.)* *Nocardia asteroides* is a ubiquitous soil saprophyte, which generally causes a bacterial infection of the lung. The reservoir of *Hantavirus* is primarily the deer mouse. There has been no well-documented human-to-human transmission of this virus. Hantaviral pulmonary syndrome is caused by the Sin Nombre virus. It was responsible for the outbreak in 1993 in the Southwest United States. The case fatality rate for this disease can be as high as 40 to 50%.

Cattle, pigs, sheep, horses, reindeer, and goats are the main reservoirs of brucellosis. A systemic disease in humans, brucellosis may be acquired from raw milk or cheese from infected animals. It is also an occupational disease of farmers, abattoir workers, veterinarians, and others who have contact with animals that may be infected. Important economic losses can be caused by brucellosis in domestic animals.

Enterobiasis is an intestinal infection with the pinworm, *Enterobius vermicularis.* The most common symptom is anal itching, particularly at night. There is no animal reservoir, but infective eggs may survive in household dust for up to 2 weeks; hence careful daily sweeping or vacuuming for a few days after treatment may prevent reinfestation. Most transmission occurs by hand from anus to mouth from the same or another person.

The definite host for *Toxoplasma gondii* is the cat and other felines. The sexual stage of its life cycle takes place in the intestinal tract of the cat. Infections during the first trimester of pregnancy can lead to severe congenital malformations. Cerebral toxoplasmosis is a common opportunistic infection in AIDS patients.

A reminder of some definitions: *host*—a human or living animal that provides the environment for an organism to grow; can be definite/primary (where the organism attains maturity), intermediate/secondary (where the organism is in larval or asexual state), or transport (where the organism is alive but does not undergo development). *Reservoir*—any person, animal, arthropod, soil, or substance where an infectious organism lives and multiplies, on which it depends for primary survival, and through which it can be transmitted to a susceptible host.

225–227. The answers are 225-d, 226-b, 227-c. (*Chin, 17/e, pp 41, 493, 537.*) St. Louis encephalitis is caused by a virus in the flavivirus family, one of a group of *arthropod-borne* "arbo" viruses. The disease is transmitted by the bite of an infected mosquito. The viruses are difficult to culture; the diagnosis is generally suspected clinically and confirmed serologically. Control of the arboviral encephalitides requires control of the insect vector—in this instance, elimination of breeding grounds for mosquitoes, destruction of larvae, screening of sleeping and living quarters, and application of residual insecticides.

Unlike other species of salmonella, *Salmonella typhi*, the cause of typhoid fever, is found only in human beings; there is no animal reservoir. *S. typhi* is excreted in the feces of human carriers. Therefore, control of the disease primarily requires adequate sanitation. Sporadic cases continue to occur in the United States; these should be investigated by public health authorities, and the actual or probable source of the infection should be identified.

Immunization with tetanus toxoid is the best means of protection against tetanus. Since the causative organism is a normal inhabitant of the intestine of many animals, including human beings, the need for immunization will persist in spite of the present rarity of the disease.

228–230. The answers are 228-a, 229-e, 230-b. (*Chin, 17/e, pp 398–388, 165–166, 70–71, 491, 302, 346.*) Most cases of botulism in the United States are food-borne and the result of inadequately heated food before home canning. Honey has also been identified as a source and should not be fed to infants. Symptoms are caused by the botulinum neurotoxin. The initial symptoms described are followed by the development of flaccid paralysis. Fever is generally absent. Botulism can also be the result of wound contamination.

Tetanus is characterized by painful muscular contractions, mainly of the masseter and neck muscles, and abdominal rigidity. General spasms occur secondary to sensory stimuli. Most cases occur in persons older than 20 years of age. Acute disease is caused by an endotoxin of the tetanus bacillus, which grows anaerobically at the site of injury.

Polio is characterized by severe muscles pains, fever, stiffness of neck and back, and asymmetrical flaccid paralysis. It is a viral infection that occurs in the gastrointestinal tract. Actually, most cases of polio (90%) are inapparent or present as nonspecific fever. Up to 1% of patients may present with aseptic meningitis.

Patients with diphtheria present with sore throat, asymmetrical grayish-white membrane on the pharynx, and nasal discharge. Patients can develop neuropathies similar to Guillain-Barré syndrome. *Haemophilus B* would present as a bacterial meningitis with fever, vomiting, lethargia, and meningeal irritation.

The neurological symptoms of Lyme disease can occur within weeks or months after the appearance of erythematus migrans (EM). They are often nonspecific and can present as facial palsy, ataxia, and chorea.

231–232. The answers are 231-c, 232-e. *(Chin, 17/e, pp 402, 332–333. CDC, MMWR 47[RR-8], 1998. USPS Task Force, 2/e, p lxii.)* The CDC issues recommendations for immunization against poliomyelitis. The Western hemisphere was certified to be free of indigenous wild polio virus in 1994 as a result of massive vaccination efforts with the oral polio vaccine. World-wide eradication seems feasible by the year 2000. The only cases of paralytic poliomyelitis (PP) in the United States are vaccine-associated, secondary to immunization with live vaccine or to a contact with a person who recently received the live vaccine. The risk of developing PP following the first oral dose of OPV is 1/750,000, and 1/2.4 million overall. Since the risk is the greatest for the first dose, the Advisory Committee on Immunization Practices (ACIP) has recommended a sequential vaccination schedule consisting of one dose of IPV at 2 months and another at 4 months, and effective January 2000, followed by a dose of IPV at 12 to 18 months and another at 4 to 6 years. A dose of MMR is recommended at 12 to 15 months and another at 4 to 6 years. Three doses of hepatitis B vaccine are recommended at birth, 1 month, and 6 months; or birth to 2 months, 1 to 2 months later, and at 6 to 18 months. Varicella vaccine is recommended at 12 to 18 months or for any susceptible child.

ENVIRONMENTAL AND OCCUPATIONAL HEALTH

Questions

DIRECTIONS: Each item below contains a question or incomplete statement followed by suggested responses. Select the **one best** response to each question.

233. Which etiological agent was responsible for most cases of illness due to waterborne-disease outbreaks in the United States in the 1990s?

a. *Salmonella enteritidis* (serotype typhimurium)
b. *Giardia lamblia*
c. *Campylobacter jejuni*
d. *Cryptosporidium parvum*
e. *Shigella sonnei*

234. The most important risk factor for heat-related illness is

a. Age over 65
b. Age under 1
c. History of prior heat stroke
d. Low socioeconomic status
e. Obesity

235. Following an accident in a nuclear laboratory, some workers were exposed to 300 rem (3 Sievert) of radiation. They are immediately sent to your emergency department. Which of the following effects will most likely occur among the majority of these workers?

a. Bone marrow depression
b. Neurovascular syndrome
c. Gastrointestinal syndrome
d. Cardiovascular syndrome
e. No detectable physiological effect

236. The Haddon matrix is used for assessing interventions for the prevention of

a. Water pollution
b. Air pollution
c. Radiation exposure
d. Injury
e. Toxic substance exposure

237. Which of the following pure tone audiograms best represents mild noise-induced hearing loss?

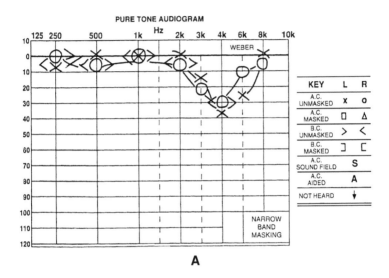

A

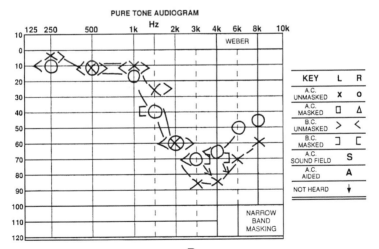

B

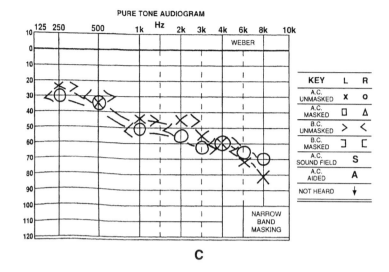

C

D

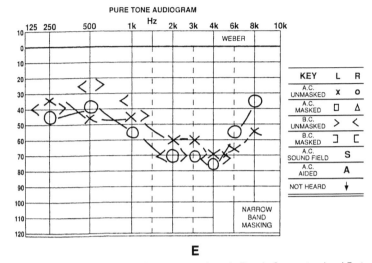

E

(Audiograms reproduced, with permission, from LaDou J., *Occupational and Environmental Medicine*, 2nd ed., Stamford, CT, Appleton & Lange, 1997: pp 125–129.)

238. The most effective means of preventing trichinosis in humans is

a. Cooking pork to reach a internal temperature of at least 40°C (104°F)
b. Proper disposal of hog feces
c. Prohibiting feeding garbage to hogs
d. Testing hogs with *Trichinella* antigen prior to slaughter
e. Freezing pork at 10°F

239. Which engineered water purification system is the most effective for the elimination of *Cryptosporidium parvum*?

a. Flocculation
b. Sedimentation
c. Disinfection
d. Boiling
e. Filtration

240. The major environmental source of lead absorbed in the human blood stream in adults is

a. Air
b. Water
c. Lead-based paint
d. Food
e. Soil

241. You are asked to evaluate the working environment in a manufacturing plant processing metal parts. In one area of the mill, where such parts are flattened, the sound level is measured at 85 dB. The workers responsible for this process are exposed to this sound for the entire 8-hour shift. The most appropriate intervention for this level of sound is

a. None. This level of sound is below the level at which OSHA regulations apply
b. A hearing conservation program
c. A shutdown of the manufacture until the level of sound is reduced
d. A shutdown only of the process area where the sound is 85 dB or higher
e. Enforcement of hearing protective devices for all exposed workers

Items 242–244

A 42-year-old welder is brought in the emergency room complaining of a sore throat, headache, and myalgias. He also started feeling a tightness in the chest and shortness of breath. He works in an electroplating operation brazing and cutting metals. Pulmonary function tests reveal a reduced forced expiratory volume. The chest x-ray is normal.

242. Which of the following exposures is the most likely cause of the worker's symptoms?

a. Lead
b. Mercury
c. Chromium
d. Copper
e. Cadmium

243. The most likely source of absorption is

a. Lung
b. Skin
c. Mucous membranes
d. Gastrointestinal
e. Open sores

244. Which of the following should be used to treat acute exposure?

a. EDTA
b. Pralidoxime
c. Dimercaprol
d. Acetylcysteine
e. Atropine

245. Toxicology is the study of adverse effects of chemicals on living organisms. Which of the following occurrences would be indicative of the most important nonthreshold effect in humans?

a. Infertility
b. Paralysis
c. Adenocarcinoma
d. Neutropenia
e. Cirrhosis

246. What proportion of cancers in humans is estimated to be the result of environmental factors?

a. 10%
b. 25%
c. 50%
d. 75%
e. 90%

Items 247–249

A 34-year-old woman is brought in from a sporting event complaining of headache, nausea, and weakness. She had been jogging outside in sunny weather where the temperature was 90° Fahrenheit with a relative humidity of 70%. She had started a training program two weeks before. She is hyperventilating, her skin is moist, and her core body temperature is 38.8° Celsius.

247. She most likely suffers from

a. Sunstroke
b. Heat cramps
c. Heat exhaustion
d. Heat stroke
e. Heat syncope

248. The most appropriate cooling measure for this patient is

a. Immersion in ice-water bath
b. Iced gastric lavage
c. Ice packs to groin, axilla, and neck
d. Evaporative cooling
e. Cool and shaded environment

249. In addition to proper hydration, rest, and attention to heat index guidelines, she should be advised to avoid reexposure to heat for at least

a. 1 day
b. 1 week
c. 2 weeks
d. 3 weeks
e. 4 weeks

250. Which of the following tests is the most frequently used rapid screening test to assess mutagenicity/carcinogenicity of a chemical substance?

a. Ames test
b. Mammalian mutation assay
c. Unscheduled DNA assay
d. Cell transformation assay
e. Cytogenetic assay

251. A migrant farm worker is brought to the clinic at 2:00 P.M. complaining of blurred vision, salivation, nausea, and diarrhea. He had been working in the fields since 6:00 A.M. in hot and humid weather. The examination reveals the following findings: heart rate of 50 per minute, respiration 20 per minute, profuse perspiration, and miosis. The most effective initial intervention with this worker is

a. Rapid administration of intravenous fluid
b. Evaporative cooling
c. Atropine
d. Observation only
e. Epinephrine

252. Which of the following waste management methods is the preferred method of waste control?

a. Waste minimization
b. Incineration
c. Recycling
d. Physical treatment
e. Biological treatment

253. Commercial airline pilots have higher exposures to which type of radiation compared to the general population?

a. Alpha particles
b. Beta particles
c. Gamma rays
d. Cosmic rays
e. X-rays

254. Radioactive waste is best disposed by

a. Physical treatment
b. Incineration
c. Landfill
d. Injection wells
e. Chemical treatment

255. Which of the following is responsible for the largest proportion of domestic water use?

a. Bathing
b. Drinking
c. Laundry
d. Toilet flushing
e. Dishwashing

256. On a hot summer day in a large urban center located in the southwestern United States, an emergency room department reports an increase in admissions for asthma in children and young adults, but not among patients suffering from chronic bronchitis or ischemic heart disease. The most likely air pollutant responsible for the exacerbation of asthma is

a. CO
b. Ozone
c. Nitrogen dioxide
d. Particulate matter
e. Lead

257. A 42-year-old welder presents to employee health services complaining of tearing eye pain and photophobia. A photokeratoconjunctivitis is diagnosed. The most likely cause of this condition is

a. Infrared radiation
b. Visible radiation
c. Ultraviolet radiation A
d. Magnetic radiation
e. Ultraviolet radiation B

258. Which of the following physical characteristics of water is the most important impediment to disinfection?

a. Color
b. Viscosity
c. Turbidity
d. Density
e. Temperature

259. Which of the following residential environmental pollutants is the leading cause of lung cancer?

a. Radon
b. Tobacco smoke
c. Asbestos
d. Formaldehyde
e. Sulfur oxide

260. Which of the following minerals is responsible for "hard water"?

a. Lead
b. Copper
c. Iron
d. Sulfur
e. Manganese

261. A 28-year-old woman presents with nausea, vomiting, and diarrhea. She has no fever. Her history reveals that she attended a reception about six hours ago. She ate roast beef with gravy, salad, and had cream-filled pastries for dessert. Prevention of this food-borne illness could have been achieved by

a. Freezing the food
b. Heating the food to 140° Fahrenheit
c. Proper hand washing by food handlers
d. Proper cleaning of contaminated surfaces
e. Control of flies

262. A 50-year-old textile worker presents to your office for his periodic health examination. He has no complaints. Review of history reveals that he has been working for over 25 years at the same company. His work consists of preparing dyes. Which of the following tests would be appropriate in this setting?

a. A chest x-ray
b. A brain computed tomography (CT) scan
c. Liver function tests
d. A complete blood count
e. A urinalysis

263. A 30-year-old patient presents at an evening walk-in clinic after work complaining of chills, fever, and malaise of acute onset. He started coughing and feeling out of breath late in the afternoon. Inspiratory crackles are present on chest auscultation. The chest x-ray is normal. The complete blood count reveals 12,000 WBC with 70% PMNs. His past medical history is benign. No one else in the household is sick. He says some of his coworkers have a cold. He works in a pet shop in the bird section. He is not taking any medication. He states he had a similar episode a few weeks ago that resolved after a few days of rest at home. The most appropriate management is to prescribe

a. Rest, fluid, and antipyretics
b. Amantadine
c. Doxycycline
d. Prednisone
e. Erythromycin

Items 264–265

A 45-year-old quarry worker presents with a history of progressive nonproductive cough and dyspnea. He has no fever or weight loss. The complete blood count is normal. The chest x-ray is as follows.

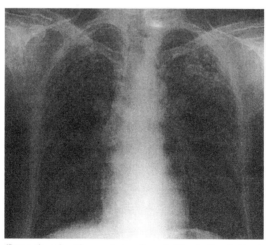

(Reproduced, with permission, from LaDou J., *Occupational and Environmental Medicine*, 2nd ed., Stamford, CT, Appleton & Lange, 1997: 320.)

264. The most likely diagnosis is

a. Caplan's syndrome
b. Silicosis
c. Asbestosis
d. Byssinosis
e. Sarcoidosis

265. He is at highest risk of developing

a. Lung cancer
b. Tuberculosis
c. Cryptococcosis
d. Chronic bronchitis
e. Emphysema

266. Biological oxygen demand (BOD) measures the total organic content of water based on the consumption of oxygen in a sample at 20° Celsius over five days. A consumption of 10 to 20 mg of O_2 per liter most likely represents a sample from

a. Treated freshwater
b. Untreated freshwater
c. Treated sewage
d. Domestic sewage
e. Industrial wastewater

267. Which of the following factors of air travel is most likely to adversely impact a patient with cardiopulmonary disease?

a. Immobility
b. Cabin air quality
c. Barometric pressure
d. Temperature
e. Humidity

268. Which of the following smokers has the highest risk of developing lung cancer?

a. An asbestos worker
b. A uranium miner
c. A coal worker
d. A textile worker
e. A sandblaster

Items 269–270

A 30-year-old man has been planning a two-week mountain-climbing trip with three other colleagues. He is in good health. He has been exercising regularly for many months in anticipation of the trip. They will be climbing to a maximum altitude of 8,500 feet. He is planning on leaving the next day.

269. When reaching the summit, this patient is at highest risk of developing

a. Headache, nausea, and sleep disturbances
b. Cough, tachypnea, and rales
c. Headache, ataxia, and altered mental status
d. Abdominal pain, flatulence, and diarrhea
e. Leg pain and swelling

270. In addition to recommending a slow ascent, prophylaxis for this patient could include

a. Nifedipine
b. Furosemide
c. Acetazolamide
d. Dexamethasone
f. Erythropoietine

271. The most important risk factor for motor vehicle injury is

a. High speed
b. Lack of use of vehicle restraints
c. Driving at night
d. Decreased vehicle size
e. Alcohol ingestion

272. Which of the following diseases is found almost exclusively among persons who have worked with or have been exposed to asbestos?

a. Bronchogenic carcinoma
b. Byssinosis
c. Pleural mesothelioma
d. Laryngeal carcinoma
e. Emphysema

273. The industry that has the highest accidental death rate in the United States is

a. Manufacturing
b. Construction
c. Mining and quarrying
d. Transportation and public utilities
e. Service

274. Following a boating accident at sea, victims are rescued by the Coast Guard and are immediately rushed for emergency medical care. Persons who were rescued from the water are more likely to experience hypothermia than those exposed only to cold air. The most likely mechanism is

a. Vasodilation
b. Thermal conductivity
c. Loss of protective barriers
d. Head injury
e. Exhaustion from efforts to stay afloat

275. During a diving expedition to explore sunken ships, one of the divers starts to experience light-headedness, dizziness, ataxia, and nausea after reaching 110 feet in depth. Which of the following is the most likely diagnosis?

a. Nitrogen narcosis
b. Barotrauma
c. Vertigo
d. Barosinusitis
e. Bends

276. Which of the following substances is causally associated with pneumoconiosis?

a. Sulfur oxides
b. Nitrogen oxides
c. Oil fumes
d. Dust particles
e. Cigarette smoke

277. Some agents have been found to be neurotoxic to the fetus and affect pregnancy outcomes. At which of the following periods will the fetus be particularly susceptible to neurotoxic substances?

a. 3 to 16 weeks
b. 6 to 9 weeks
c. 4 to 8 weeks
d. 3 to 6 weeks
e. 7 to 9 weeks

278. A couple presents to the infertility clinic because of inability to conceive for over one year. A semen analysis on the male reveals oligospermia. He works for a company that manufactures storage batteries. A blood level should be obtained for which of the following agents?

a. Chromium
b. Nickel
c. Lead
d. Antimony
e. Boron

279. Different reproductive outcomes can be used in studies examining the effect of exposure to a particular potentially toxic substance. Which of the following studies is most likely to be subject to bias?

a. A study examining an association with early spontaneous abortion
b. A study examining an association with late spontaneous abortion
c. A study examining an association with congenital anomalies
d. A study examining an association with preterm birth
e. A study examining an association with low birth weight

280. A large explosion occurs at a construction site during excavation. None of the workers appear injured. Some of them were exposed to sound pressure levels of 190 dB. Which of the following is the most likely outcome for these workers?

a. Temporary tinnitus
b. Temporary conductive hearing loss
c. Permanent conductive hearing loss
d. Temporary sensorineural loss
e. Permanent sensorineural loss

281. Ergonomics is also called human factors engineering, and examines ways to adapt the working environment to ensure a safe and productive workplace. Which of the following factors is the most important to improve the physical design of a sedentary job?

a. Maintaining a static position
b. Maintaining a standing position
c. Eliminating the waist motion
d. Installing a soft floor
e. Maintaining a static holding position

282. Which of the following methods is most effective in reducing radon levels in homes and buildings?

a. Maintaining a sealed environment and recirculating air
b. Repairing cracks in the foundation
c. Keeping windows open
d. Venting air on the upper floors
e. Insulating the basement

283. "Hard water" has been associated with which of the following beneficial health effects?

a. Decrease in cardiovascular disease
b. Decrease in colorectal cancer
c. Decrease in lung cancer
d. Decrease in anemia
e. Decrease in osteoporosis

284. A 50-year-old presents with dyspnea on exertion, without cough or chest pain. He has no history of asthma, chronic bronchitis, or heart disease. He does not smoke. He is employed in the aircraft industry and his work consists of producing metal alloys. His chest x-ray reveals small, rounded, and irregular opacities. Pulmonary function tests show decreased diffusion. The Kveim for sarcoidosis is negative. The most likely etiologic agent responsible for these findings is

a. X-rays
b. Beryllium
c. Tantalum
d. Uranium
e. Carbon dioxide

285. Vibration, low temperatures, repetition, and force can all contribute to the development of repetitive motion disorders. Which of the following industries is associated with the highest rate of disorders associated with repeated trauma?

a. Grocery stores
b. Manufacturing electronic equipment
c. Computer manufacturing
d. Meat-packing plants
e. Poultry slaughtering

286. You are employed by a city health department and oversee the quality of recreational waters in your area. There is a lake with a beach that is very crowded during the summer. Which of the following organisms would you quantitatively measure on a regular basis to assess the safety of the water?

a. Coliform
b. *Escherichia coli*
c. *Giardia lamblia*
d. Norwalk virus
e. *Salmonella*

Items 287–289

Match the following events with the most appropriate legislative act.

a. Medical Waste Tracking Act 1988
b. Comprehensive Environmental Response, Compensation and Liabilities Act 1980
c. Resource Conservation and Recovery Act 1976
d. National Environmental Protection Act 1970
e. Federal Insecticide, Fungicide and Rodenticide Act 1972
f. Toxic Substance Control Act 1976
g. Clean Water Act 1972
h. Safe Drinking Water Act 1974
i. Clean Air Act 1970

287. Ban of the manufacturing and distribution of asbestos.

288. Ban of the use of PCBs for all but emergencies.

289. Hazardous waste site cleanup.

Items 290–293

Match the following clinical presentations with the most likely metal exposure.

a. Arsenic
b. Beryllium
c. Cadmium
d. Chromium
e. Lead
f. Manganese
g. Mercury
h. Nickel
i. Zinc

290. A worker presents with hyperkeratosis, hyperpigmentation, and anemia.

291. A worker presents with Fanconi's syndrome.

292. A worker experiences fever, chills, profuse sweating, cough, and chest pain that resolves after 48 hours.

293. A worker presents with ataxia, loss of visual fields, and auditory disturbances.

Items 294–295

Match the following clinical presentation with the most likely solvent exposure.

a. Hydrocarbons
b. Petroleum distillates
c. Alcohols
d. Glycols
e. Ketones
f. Esters
g. Phenols

294. A worker presents with optic neuropathy, blurred vision, and blindness.

295. A worker presents with hepatic and kidney necrosis.

Items 296–298

Match the following organ toxicity with the most likely exposure.

a. Arsenic
b. Carbon tetrachloride
c. Quartz
d. Coal
e. Cotton
f. Acrylic
g. DDT

296. Cardiovascular toxicity, including arrythmia, myocardial injury, and peripheral arterial occlusive disease.

297. Acute liver toxicity with necrosis (liver).

298. Chloracne (skin).

Items 299–300

For each poisoning with the agents listed below, select the appropriate treatment.

a. Pralidoxime
b. Amyl nitrite
c. Dimercaprol
d. Edetate calcium disodium
e. Acetylcysteine
f. Flumazenil

299. Parathion.

300. Mercury.

Items 301–303

Match each of the workers below with the infectious disease for which they are at risk.

a. Hepatitis B
b. Brucellosis
c. Legionnaire's disease
d. Histoplasmosis
e. Sporotrochosis

301. Butcher.

302. Air conditioner repair person.

303. Dentist.

Items 304–305

Certain substances in the occupational environment have been identified as carcinogenic agents based on epidemiologic evidence obtained in studies of exposed laboratory animals and human populations. Match each chemical agent with the human target site for cancer.

a. Liver
b. Brain
c. Bladder
d. Lung
e. Hematopoietic systems
f. Bone

304. Benzene.

305. Radium.

ENVIRONMENTAL AND OCCUPATIONAL HEALTH

Answers

233. The answer is d. *(USDHHS, MMWR 45 [SS-1], 1996.) Cryptosporidium parvum* was responsible for illness in 403,271 persons, the greatest number of cases of illness due to outbreaks of waterborne disease in the United States in the 1990s. During an outbreak in Milwaukee in 1993, an estimated 403,000 persons became ill and 4,400 were hospitalized. Although the actual number of outbreaks as opposed to number of cases is about the same for *C. parvum* and *G. lamblia,* outbreaks of *G. lamblia* caused illness in an estimated 385 persons.

234. The answer is a. *(LaDou, 2/e, pp 144–145.)* Older adults over the age of 65 are particularly at risk of death due to heat-related illness because of decreased response of the cardiovascular system during hot weather. Very young children under the age of 1 are also at risk, but less than older persons. Heat-related illness is seen more frequently in lower-socioeconomic areas, presumably because of no access to air conditioning and good ventilation and because of higher temperatures in urban areas ("heat islands"). Obesity and prior history of heat stroke also increase the risk, but to a much lesser degree than older age. Drugs that inhibit sweat production, cause dehydration, and reduce cutaneous blood flow (atropine, antidepressants, diuretics, etc.) also increase susceptibility to heat.

235. The answer is a. *(LaDou, 2/e, pp 159–161.)* Disturbances begin to occur at exposures above 100 rem. Following an acute exposure to 100 to 200 rem of ionizing radiation, mild hematopoietic disturbances may occur (5% at 100 rem and 50% at 200 rem) after a few weeks, which only warrant surveillance. Some patients may have vomiting three hours after the exposure. Between 200 and 600 rem, more severe hematopoietic disturbances will occur, with a peak at 4 to 6 weeks, requiring transfusions, antibiotics, and hematopoietic growth factors. Patients will vomit within two hours. Extreme disturbances will occur after an acute exposure of 600 to 1000 rem, with a high case fatality rate (80 to 100% within two months). Vomiting will occur within one hour. All patients with exposures above 1000 rem will die, with early onset (1 to 14 days depending on exposure) of gastrointestinal syndrome (diarrhea, fever, and electrolyte disturbances) and central nervous system problems dominating the clinical picture.

236. The answer is d. (*Christoffel, 1999, pp 30–33.*) This is a systematic approach to injury prevention developed by William Haddon Jr. of the New York State Department. The matrix categorizes interventions as modifying the host, agent, and environment either before, at the time of, or after the event.

237. The answer is a. (*LaDou, 2/e, pp 123–130.*) These are examples of audiograms showing response to pure tone in air conduction (A.C) and bone conduction (B.C). Thresholds of hearing are expressed in decibels (the y axis). Because loud noise may stimulate the contralateral ear, masking the opposite ear is necessary. When both air and bone conduction are decreased, there is a neurosensorial loss. Conductive losses are characterized by a gap between air and bone conduction where the air-conduction loss exceeds the bone loss. Noise-induced hearing loss is typically most pronounced at 4000 Hz. As the deficit becomes more severe, hearing begins deteriorating at less that 4000 Hz (audiogram B). Hearing loss due to noise is *sensorineural:* air conduction will be better than bone conduction with the Rinne test (tuning fork). Aging can also cause a sensorineural hearing deficit (presbycusis), but the loss generally increases with the frequency: deficit at 8000 Hz will be more pronounced than at 4000 Hz, and the audiogram shows a slow descending curve (audiogram C). Middle-ear or external-ear dysfunction will cause a discrepency between bone and air conduction, as illustrated in audiogram D. Nonorganic hearing loss (that is "faking" hearing loss) can usually be discovered by audiogram E: persons will tend to claim gradual hearing difficulties with poor correlation with speech discrimination. There will also often be test-retest variability.

238. The answer is c. (*Chin, 17/e, p 510.*) Infection of hogs with nematodes of the genus *Trichinella* can be prevented by ensuring that all garbage and offal fed to the hogs are heat-treated to destroy the cysts or, preferably, by using feed devoid of animal meat, such as grain. Prohibition of marketing of garbage-fed hogs is easier to enforce than inspection to ensure that all garbage is properly cooked. The disease is transmitted by ingestion of larvae in hog skeletal muscle, not by hog feces. Thorough cooking of pork and pork products so that all the meat reaches at least 71°C (160°F) destroys the encysted larvae. Freezing pork also destroys the larvae if adequate time-temperature schedules are followed. In order to be effective, freezing must be done at −15°C (−5°F) for 30 days if the piece of meat is 15 cm in thickness or less.

239. The answer is e. *(LaDou, 2/e, pp 735–739.)* Slow sand, rapid granular, or membrane filtration is the most effective water treatment method to remove *Cryptosporidium* cysts, as they are not destroyed by disinfection. Flocculation is used to help form large floc particles from particulate matter including bacteria which can then can be more easily removed. Sedimentation, through gravity, makes particulates including bacteria settle to the bottom of a tank. Flocculation and sedimentation do not effectively remove cysts. It is important to note that high water turbidity may affect the ability of filtration to remove the parasite, and that filtration may not always afford absolute protection. Boiling is not an engineered water sanitation process, but it is the simplest effective method to prevent *Cryptosporidium parvum* infections if drinking water is contaminated or has not been treated adequately. The water intended for drinking should be boiled for 1 min. Immunosuppressed persons, such as those with HIV, are particularly at risk of severe infections (see Chapter 2).

240. The answer is a. *(LaDou, 2/e, pp 649–651.)* Although most lead intake in humans is from ingestion of lead-contaminated food (about 0.1 mg of lead is ingested daily per person), the amount of lead that is absorbed after inhalation of lead-contaminated air is of greater significance because up to 50% of inhaled lead, compared with only as much as 10% of ingested lead, is absorbed and circulated through the blood. Because modern building codes require the replacement of lead domestic water-supply pipes with those made of copper or galvanized iron, drinking water has become a decreasing source of lead poisoning. The intake of lead through ingestion of lead-based paint is mainly a problem with children. Gastrointestinal absorption of lead appears to be more efficient in children, while pulmonary absorption is more efficient in adults.

241. The answer is b. *(LaDou, 2/e, pp 132–134.)* Exposures of 85 dB or more for 8 hours a day or more require the implementation of a hearing conservation program (HCP) under OSHA (Occupational Safety and Health

Administration) regulation. This program includes noise monitoring, engineering controls, administrative control, worker education, selection and use of hearing protection devices (HPD), and periodic audiometric evaluations. Engineering controls where possible are always the preferred method of controlling sound levels. Administrative controls include reducing the amount of time the worker is exposed to high levels of sound. This is often difficult to achieve and requires constant oversight to ensure implementation. Hearing devices must be able to bring the level of sound to 90 dB or less, the permissable exposure level for sound. However, workers may not always wear these devices. At levels of sound below 90 dB, OSHA requires that HPD be made available to workers. At level 90 or above, HPD must be provided and proper use must be enforced by the employer.

242–244. The answers are 242-e, 243-a, 244-a. (*LaDou, 2/e, pp 209, 413–415.*) Acute exposure to mercury results in cough, inflammation of the oral cavity, and gastrointestinal symptoms. Renal injury is of particular concern. Neurological symptoms can later occur. Mercury is often used in the manufacturing of control instruments (such as thermometers). Dimercaprol is used for treatment. Copper toxicity (in the United States) is primarily due to accidental ingestion or suicide attempts and leads to intravascular hemolysis and methemoglobinemia. No specific treatment exists. The initial symptoms associated with acute exposure (ingestion or inhalation) of lead are primarily gastrointestinal (abdominal cramps). Encephalopathy can follow. Lead is used intensively in the production of storage batteries. Chromium is used in plating. Acute exposure results in irritation of eyes, nose, and throat with epistaxis. Chromium is a known carcinogen (lung cancer). Dermatologic conditions are common among chromium workers (ulcerations with delayed healing on fingers, knuckles, and forearms) and are treated with 10% $CaNa_2$ EDTA ointment. Atropine and pralidoxime are used in the treatment of pesticide exposure (see question 251). Acetylcysteine is used for acetaminophen poisoning.

245. The answer is c. (*LaDou, 2/e, pp 176–177.*) Substances causing adverse biological effects in humans can be classified as reproductive, renal, and respiratory toxins; neurotoxins, dermatotoxins, and hepatotoxins. It is assumed that there may be some form of dose-response relationship and that there is a minimal exposure below which a toxic effect will not occur (the threshold). The absence of threshold is assumed for any substance that is carcinogenic, mutagenic, and/or teratogenic. There is no safe exposure below which no effect exists. In other words, a nonthreshold effect exists when there is no safe level of exposure to humans.

246. The answer is e. *(Wallace, 14/e, pp 914–920.)* Most cancers are caused by one or a combination of exposure(s) due to the environment or lifestyle such as tobacco smoke, radon, chemicals, asbestos, toxins, and ultraviolet light.

247–249. The answers are 247-c, 248-e, 249-a. *(LaDou, 2/e, pp 142–148.)* Heat stroke is characterized by the presence of mental status changes and a core body temperature of more than 39° Celsius. Cardiovascular collapse will occur if not treated immediately as the body temperature may reach up to 41.1° Celsius. This is a medical emergency requiring IV hydration and rapid cooling: cool water or isopropyl alcohol 70% on the body with fanning, sponge baths, ice packs on the groin/axilla/neck, and/or iced gastric lavage until the core body temperature drops to 39° Celsius. Patients should be advised to avoid heat exposure for at least 4 weeks because hypersensitivity to heat may persist for a long period of time after an episode of heat stroke. Heat cramps are characterized by painful muscle cramps along with some nausea and vomiting. The core body temperature is normal. This is caused by sodium depletion due to sweating: the patient should be placed in a cool environment and hydrated with a balanced salt solution. Rest for at least 1 to 3 days is recommended. Heat syncope is a sudden loss of consciousness due to vasodilation secondary to heat. Heat exhaustion is what this patient is experiencing. She should be placed in a cool and shaded environment. This patient should also receive hydration and salt replenishment with IV fluids. Milder cases can be treated with oral hydration. At least 1 day of rest is recommended after heat exhaustion. Heat index guidelines are developed by the National Weather Service and predict risk of heat-related disorders based on ambient heat and humidity.

250. The answer is a. *(LaDou, 2/e, pp 241–242.)* All the tests listed can be used to screen substances for mutagenesis and carcinogenesis, that is, their ability to interact with genetic material and DNA. The Ames test is the most commonly used rapid screening test and is a bacterial mutation assay. It tests for the reversion of a histidine-requiring *Salmonella typhimurium* mutant to the wild type. It is very sensitive to DNA damage. The other tests are more sophisticated, take more time, and are more expensive.

251. The answer is c. *(LaDou, 2/e, pp 547–554.)* The clinical signs are not consistent with heat-related illness, but rather poisoning with the commonly used pesticide carbamate. Symptoms are related to the inhibition of cholinesterase. Mild symptoms are characterized by muscarinic signs and symptoms. Atropine blocks the effect of acetylcholine at the muscarinic receptors.

252. The answer is a. *(Wallace, 14/e, p 768.)* Minimizing waste is the best approach to controlling the problem by reducing the amount of waste generated. Recycling, when possible, is the next best method, followed by incineration when appropriate (organic compounds can be reduced to water, carbon dioxide, and heat). Physical treatment is most commonly used for water treatment (sedimentation, filtration, flocculation). Chemical treatment can be used to transform hazardous substances into less-toxic ones. Biological treatment can be used to treat industrial wastewater, a major source of waste.

253. The answer is d. *(Wallace, 14/e, p 619.)* Natural background radiation (terrestrial and cosmic radiation, naturally occurring radionuclides) is the most important source of radiation exposure for all humans. Radiation from manufactured origins accounts for only 20% of all radiation exposure. Terrestrial radiation, consisting of gamma rays (average exposure: 40–50 mrem per year), varies with geography, and cosmic radiation due to cosmic rays (average exposure: 40–50 mrem per year) increases with altitude. Air travel increases exposure and aircrews have five times greater exposure than the general population. Alpha radiation has very limited penetration because of the large size of the particles and is completely absorbed by the outer layer of the skin. However, hazard occurs when these particles enter the body and irradiate living tissue (radon daughters that are inhaled). Beta particles are all internal hazards, but external exposure can be stopped by one inch of water. Cosmic rays are more penetrating than gamma rays. X-rays are indistinguishable from gamma rays, except for their origin (synthetic versus natural terrestrial).

254. The answer is c. *(Wallace, 14/e, p 768.)* Landfills are used to dispose of nonliquid waste only. This is the only method of disposing of radioactive waste safely. Other methods are used to dispose of nonradioactive waste (see answer to question 252).

255. The answer is d. *(Wallace, 14/e, p 738.)* Which is why laws were enacted to set a maximum limit on the amount of water a toilet can use for each flush. About 40% of water is taken up by flushing, 30% by bathing, 15% by laundry, 5% by drinking/cooking, and 5% by dishwashing.

256. The answer is b. *(LaDou, 2/e, pp 707–712.)* The major air pollutants are particulates, sulfur oxides, carbon monoxide, oxides of nitrogen, hydrocarbons, lead, and ozone. The latter is formed by sunlight irradiating an atmosphere containing hydrocarbons and oxides of nitrogen, and has been associated with Southern California smog. It has primarily been linked to an exacerbation of asthma. Hydrocarbons are precursors of smog. Carcinogenicity is debated. Oxides of nitrogen are also precursors of smog: important sources are automobiles and airplanes. They are primarily mucosal irritants and studies on respiratory effects are conflicting. Carbon monoxide, although a plentiful pollutant, is quickly transformed into carbon dioxide. Increases will aggravate coronary artery disease, precipitate myocardial infarction, and reduce exercise tolerance. Particulate matter will most severely affect persons with chronic obstructive pulmonary disease. Sulfur oxide is the most important air pollutant.

257. The answer is e. *(LaDou, 2/e, pp 152–157.)* Ultraviolet radiation covers the spectrum between visible radiation (light) and ionizing radiation (100–400 nm). Ultraviolet radiation B ranges from 280 to 315 nm, the range to which the eye is particularly sensitive and where most injuries occur. *Acute* exposure to UV of less than 315 nm results in photokeratoconjunctivitis, with symptoms appearing 6 to 12 hours after exposure. *Prolonged* exposures to UV between 295 and 320 nm can result in cataract formation. Ultraviolet A ranges from 315 to 400 nm. Injuries caused by vis-

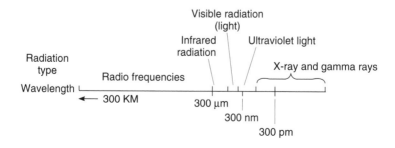

ible radiation (light), which covers the spectrum between infrared and ultraviolet radiation (400–750 nm), affect primarily the retina, which is most sensitive to blue light (eclipse blindness). Infrared light covers the spectrum between visible light and radiofrequency (750 to 3 million nm). It is given off by any material of a temperature greater than absolute zero. Thermal injury can occur with intense exposure to infrared light of less than 2000 nm and has been associated with cataract formation.

258. The answer is c. *(Wallace, 14/e, p 745.)* Turbidity is a major impediment to disinfection. Major steps in potable water treatment are sedimentation, coagulation (often alum is added to facilitate floc formation that will settle more readily) and flocculation, which get rid of 90% of the bacterial load and reduce color and turbidity (see question 239). Filtration eliminates particles which cannot be destroyed by other methods, such a cysts from *Cryptosporidium, Entamoeba hystolitica,* and *Giardia lamblia.* Finally, the water is disinfected generally with chlorine whose power is greater at lower pH. Residual levels remain in the water as it is distributed to consumers, a major advantage over ozone.

259. The answer is b. *(LaDou, 2/e, pp 246, 251–252, 656.)* Tobacco is still a leading cause of lung cancer. Radon has also been associated with lung cancer, and the combination of radon and tobacco smoke can be synergistic. Lung cancer is responsible for 20% of all asbestos-related deaths. Formaldehyde has been associated with nasopharyngeal cancers. Sulfur oxide is primarily an outdoor pollutant (see question 256).

260. The answer is e. *(Wallace, 14/e, p 744.)* So-called "hard water" is primarily due to high concentrations of calcium or manganese. Soft water can be corrosive and leach metals from pipes, especially lead.

261. The answer is c. *(Chin, 17/e, pp 203–206.)* The short incubation period and symptoms are characteristic of food poisoning due to the toxin produced by *Staphylococcus aureus.* Organisms and toxin are not destroyed by freezing. Although the organisms can be killed by heating food to 66° Celsius (150° Fahrenheit), the preformed toxin generally survives. Optimum growth of the bacteria occurs at 59° to 99° Fahrenheit (growth is inhibited at below 39° Fahrenheit), with toxin production optimal after 4 to 6 hours. The source is human skin, mouth, and nose. Proper hand washing by food handlers and excluding those with skin infections is the best way to prevent contamination.

262. The answer is e. *(LaDou, 2/e, pp 244.)* Dye workers are susceptible to bladder cancer due to exposure to β-Naphtylamine and benzidine. The most common presenting symptom will be gross hematuria or microscopic hematuria. Liver cancer has been associated with exposure to vinyl chloride while hematologic cancers are associated with radiation and benzene exposure. Occupational causes of brain cancer have not been well identified at this time.

263. The answer is a. *(LaDou, 2/e, pp 315–317. Fauci, 14/e, p 726.)* These symptoms are typical of hypersensitivity pneumonitis, which can often be confused with infectious causes such as influenza or *Mycoplasma pneumoniae*. Chest x-ray may be completely normal even in symptomatic individuals. However, typically, the chest x-ray may show bilateral reticulonodular infiltrates. The acute form is characterized by the appearance of symptoms a few hours after short-term high exposure, and resolves after a few hours or days. Treatment should primarily consist of avoiding the causative agent or wearing respiratory protective equipment. Acute episodes resolve on their own without glucocorticosteroids. Prednisone is the treatment for severe or progressive hypersensitivity pneumonitis. Psittacosis has an incubation period of 7 to 14 days, can be associated with splenomegaly (10 to 70% of cases), and the x-ray generally shows diffuse patchy infiltrates.

264–265. The answers are 264-b, 265-b. *(LaDou, 2/e, pp 320–321.)* Silicosis, a pneumoconiosis, is caused by respiratory exposure to silica, a major component of rock and sand. Patients with silicosis are at risk of mycobacterium infection, both atypical and typical. A positive PPD in a patient with chronic silicosis warrants preventive tuberculosis therapy. They are also at higher risk for fungal infections such as cryptococcosis. Asbestos increases the risk of lung cancer and mesothelioma. Byssinosis is an occupational form of asthma due to cotton dust inhalation. Caplan's syndrome may occur in coal miners who also have rheumatoid arthritis and is characterized by rapidly evolving rounded densities on chest x-rays.

266. The answer is c. *(LaDou, 2/e, p 735.)* Biological oxygen demand is a measure of organic content in water. The greater the demand, the greater the load of organic content that can be broken down, reflecting a high bacterial load. Untreated freshwater has a BOD of 2–5 mg/l, treated sewage, 10–20, domestic sewage, 200–500, and industrial sewage, >2000.

267. The answer is c. *(Fauci, 14/e [full text], p 150.)* Lower barometric pressure associated with air travel will lower the tension of oxygen in the inspired air, the alveolar oxygen tension, and arterial oxygen saturation, which could lead to an exacerbation of coronary artery disease deficiency. Immobilization for long periods of time can increase the risk of thromboembolic disease, which may be more of an issue for pregnant women. Getting up periodically to walk up and down the aisles may help alleviate this problem. The circadian rhythm will be changed due to the change in time zones and peaks of cortisol production will also vary. This can potentially affect the pathophysiology and timing of cardiac events. Cabin air quality studies have shown that the CO, CO_2, and respirable particulate levels are below OSHA standards, and that ozone levels are below the Federal Aviation Administration (FAA) standards.

268. The answer is a. *(LaDou, 2/e, pp 715–716.)* The effect of asbestos and smoking are synergistic for the development of lung cancer. Uranium workers, due to exposure to radon, will also be at greater risk, particularly if they are exposed to higher levels of radiation (a dose response relationship has been described).

269–270. The answers are 269-a, 270-c. *(Kozarsky, 1998. Ryan, 2000.)* Acute mountain sickness, as described in A, is the most common altitude illness and usually occurs in altitudes above 8000 feet (2500 m). Symptoms occur about 3 to 12 hours after reaching that level. It will resolve spontaneously after 5 to 7 days at altitude. Acetazolamide 125 to 250 mg every 8 to 12 hours starting 24 hours before the ascent and to be continued for 2 days at altitude or 500 mg SR tablet every 24 hours and continued for 2 days at altitude may alleviate symptoms. Dexamethasone 4 mg every 6 to 12 hours is reserved for those intolerant/allergic to Acetazolamide or for treatment of more serious altitude sickness. High-altitude pulmonary edema can occur (1 to 2% of individuals) at altitudes of over 10,000 feet. Symptoms of tachypnea and dyspnea with rales start 2 to 4 days before reaching that altitude. They can be rapidly fatal if not treated. Treatment consists of rapid descent and nifedipine. High-altitude cerebral edema occurs occasionally (less than 1% of persons) at altitudes above 15,000 feet, but may occur as low as 9,000 feet in susceptible individuals. Symptoms are described in answer C for question 269. Rapid descent and dexamethasone is the required treatment. Persons may also experience abdominal bloating due to the expansion of gas in the bowel, but it is not associated with diarrhea.

271. The answer is e. *(Christoffel, pp 74–75.)* At least two-fifths of all motor vehicle deaths are alcohol-related. Some statistics report 50%. A motor vehicle crash–related death is most likely to occur with a young male, at night, on a rural road in a single-vehicle crash. Most crashes occur in the summer. Use of a larger, more crashworthy vehicle and use of restraints such as seatbelts reduce the incidence of death related to the accident.

272. The answer is c. *(LaDou, 2/e, pp 244, 254–256.)* Asbestos has been linked to lung cancer, the most common neoplasia associated with this exposure, colon cancer, and kidney cancer. Pleural and peritoneal mesotheliomas are particular to asbestos exposure. Lung cancers have also been linked to arsenic, beryllium, cadmium, chromium, and mustard gas.

273. The answer is c. *(LaDou, 2/e, p 4.)* Mining and quarrying is the most dangerous industry in the United States. Construction is next, followed by agriculture. A shift toward a service industry and away from manufacturing jobs, which involve equipment and machinery, and safer work environments have resulted in overall declines in occupational injury and deaths.

274. The answer is b. *(Wallace, 14/e, p 615.)* Conduction is the principal source of heat loss during cold-water immersion. Thermal conductivity of water is 25 times that of air. Alcohol can precipitate heat loss in both air or water immersion due to the vasodilation it produces. Exhaustion may also be a contributing factor to heat loss in water versus air.

275. The answer is a. *(LaDou, 2/e, pp 163–166.)* Nitrogen narcosis is due to increased partial pressure of nitrogen in the nervous system and symptoms are analogous to alcohol intoxication. Barotrauma (barosinusitis, middle ear or barotitis media) is due to the mechanical effects of expansion and contraction of gases when pressure differences exist between the body cavities and the environment. These two syndromes are manifestations of *compression* sickness occurring during descent. "The bends" (so called because the person can be stooped because of severe joint pain) are a form of *decompression* sickness (also called caisson disease) due to inadequate elimination of dissolved gas after a dive, affecting the skin and joints. Decompression sickness can occur either after a too rapid ascent from a dive below 9 meters or a sudden pressure loss at altitudes above 7000 feet.

276. The answer is d. *(LaDou, 2/e, pp 320–323.)* Pneumoconiosis, a fibrosing disease of the lungs, usually occurs as a result of occupational exposure to air that contains particulate matter, especially mineral dust. Anthracosis, silicosis, asbestosis, and berylliosis are among the more than 30 forms of pneumoconioses that have been described in the literature. Sulfur oxides, nitrogen oxides, oil fumes, and cigarette smoke are likely to cause acute bronchospasm or to exacerbate preexisting diseases such as chronic bronchitis and emphysema.

277. The answer is a. *(LaDou, 2/e, p 380.)* Susceptibility of the central nervous system extends beyond 8 weeks, contrary to most other organ development. The eyes and the ears are usually not susceptible to teratogens. Enhanced susceptibility of the external genitalia starts at a later period than most other organs (about 7 weeks) and extends to 9 weeks. The heart is more susceptible between 3 to 6 weeks.

278. The answer is c. *(LaDou, 2/3, p 398.)* Carbon disulfide, chloroprene, estrogens, excessive heat, lead, and ionizing radiation have all been strongly linked to oligospermia. Exposure to lead can occur during the manufacturing of storage batteries. Chromium, nickel, and antimony levels are measured in urine, but are not associated with oligospermia.

279. The answer is a. *(LaDou, 2/e, pp 383–384.)* Early spontaneous abortion (SAB) is particularly difficult to evaluate. If the study is prospective, women exposed to a particular substance who may be worried about it may seek earlier medical care, and the pregnancy will be detected earlier. Thus, more losses will be detected compared to women who present at a later time in pregnancy, as early spontaneous abortion is a relatively frequent event. Therefore, it is important to define when and how the pregnancy is diagnosed (chemical versus clinical). If a case-control study is undertaken based on medical records, some early SABs that are due to the exposure may be missed. The other outcomes mentioned can be better defined and are less subject to bias. Cohort studies are particularly well suited to examine pregnancy outcomes given the short follow-up period. However, since some of the outcomes in question can be very rare (such as congenital anomalies), case-control studies may sometimes be more appropriate.

280. The answer is b. *(LaDou, 2/e, pp 135–136.)* *Acute* exposures to sound pressure levels above 180 dB will result in a traumatic rupture of the tympanic membrane and conductive hearing loss. The rupture should repair spontaneously unless infection occurs. If the loss persists for more than three months, surgical repair is possible. Sensorineural loss is generally due to fractures or trauma to the inner ear. Mixed hearing loss can occur secondary to fractures of the temporal bone, when both the middle and the inner ear are traumatized.

281. The answer is c. *(LaDou, 2/e, pp 42–46.)* Static body and holding positions should be avoided. For instance, persons working at a computer terminal should be reminded to do a short walking task every 20 minutes. Objects can be placed on a supporting surface instead of handheld. Eliminating the waist motion such that everything needed is within arm's reach will reduce stress on back, neck, and shoulders. The less torso movement, the better.

282. The answer is b. *(Ladou, 2/e, p 656.)* Radon diffuses from rocks and soil containing uranium during radioactive decay. It can also be found in water. Since 1988, the EPA has recommended that homes below the third floor be tested for radon, which is recognized as the second leading cause of lung cancer after tobacco smoke. Homes that are sealed carry a greater risk of higher concentrations. Keeping the basement free of cracks and holes, aeration, and venting radon-laden air from beneath the foundation can all be helpful. Keeping windows open may not be a very practical solution, but can be effective.

283. The answer is a. *(Wallace, 14/e, p 744.)* Hard water requires more soap for bathing and laundering. There have been some studies that have demonstrated an inverse relationship between the hardness of water and cardiovascular mortality rates, making an argument against water softening.

284. The answer is b. *(Wallace, 14/e, p 496. Fauci, 14/e, p 1927.)* Beryllium causes a syndrome similar to sarcoidosis. Only individuals who are sensitized to the metal will develop the disease. It can also cause granulomas of the skin. Tantalum is increasingly used in alloys for the aerospace industry, but has caused few health problems. Uranium causes exposure to radon, a known carcinogen of the lung. The Kveim-Siltzbach consists of an intradermal injection of a heat-treated suspension of sarcoidosis spleen extract. A biopsy is taken at the site 4 to 6 weeks later. Patients with sarcoidosis will develop sarcoidosis-like lesions in the skin.

285. The answer is d. *(Wallace, 14/e, p 671.)* Much of the work requires cutting up carcasses on an assembly with a heavy saw and in a bent position. All of this is done in a refrigerated environment, which predisposes workers to repetitive motion disorders (RMD). The occupation has therefore all of the risk factors for developing RMD: force, repetition, cold temperature, vibration, and bad posture.

286. The answer is b. *(Wallace, 14/e, p 747.)* The Environmental Protection Agency (EPA) produced guidelines in 1986 recommending that states adopt the enterococcus or *E. coli* criterion for freshwater and the enterococcus criteria for saltwater, based on the observation that there existed a linear relationship between enterococcus and *E. coli* (but not coliforms) concentrations and swimming-associated gastrointestinal symptoms.

287–289. The answers are 287-f, 288-e, 289-b. *(Wallace, 14/e, pp 470, 587, 741, 662, 765.)* The Medical Waste Tracking Act of 1988 set requirements for separating, packaging, and labeling medical wastes and required the Agency for Toxic Substances and Disease Registry (ATSDR) to prepare a report on the health effects of medical waste. The Resource Conservation and Recovery Act (RCRA) established the first comprehensive federal regulatory program for controlling hazardous waste. The National Environmental Protection Act (NEPA) of 1970 required any federal agency proposing a project having potential adverse effects on the environment to develop an environmental impact statement. The Clean Water Act of 1972 was designed to protect recreational waters, not drinking water. The Safe Drinking Water Act of 1974 provided national drinking water standards. The Clean Air Act of 1970 is the most important federal law protecting the air we breathe, and created the national Ambient Air Quality Standards. The Federal Insecticide, Fungicide and Rodenticide Act (FIFRA) is the primary federal law for regulating the manufacture, distribution, and use of pesticides and requires that all pesticides sold or distributed in the United States be registered with the EPA.

290–293. The answers are 290-a, 291-c, 292-i, 293-g. *(LaDou, 2/e, pp 408, 412, 421, 432.)* Chronic exposure to arsenic causes the symptoms described in question 290. Acute exposure can lead to cardiovascular collapse. Beryllium can cause upper respiratory symptoms after acute exposure, and granulomas with a chronic debilitating disease (respiratory symptoms accompanied by weight loss and fatigue) after chronic exposure (berylliosis). Chronic exposure to cadmium can cause Fanconi's syndrome (only metal to cause this). Chronic exposure to chromium can lead to nasal perforation and lung cancer. Acute exposure to nickel may result in bronchospasm (inhalation) and dermatitis (skin contact). Lead exposure leads to neurological disturbances such as encephalopathy (if acute), neuropathy, and neurobehavioral changes. Chronic exposure to manganese may lead to a Parkinsonlike disease. Exposure to mercury can cause ataxia, spasticity, parethesias, and visual disturbances. The symptoms described in question 292 are often called "metal fume fever" and are typical of an acute exposure to zinc.

294–295.   The answers are 294-c, 295-g. *(LaDou, 2/e, pp 498–509.)* Remember that *all* the solvents listed will cause some form of CNS depression after *acute* exposure ("drunkenness," slurred speech, dizziness, headache). Exposure occurs by inhalation or skin absorption. They will also all cause some form of dermatitis after chronic skin exposure (cracked and erythematous skin). Chronic exposure to esters and ketones results only in dermatitis, with no other health effects demonstrated. Chronic exposure to all types of hydrocarbons and petroleum distillates results in neurobehavioral dysfunction and short-term memory loss, difficulty concentrating, fatigue. Methyl alcohol is widely used as an industrial solvent and one-third methyl alcohol is used in formaldehyde. Chronic toxicity (which can occur through inhalation) produces optic neuropathy (particular to this type of alcohol; not seen with other solvents). Only acute exposure to phenols causes the tissue destruction described in question 295. Although all solvents can potentially cause some form of hepatotoxicity if exposure is high and long enough, halogen and nitro group are particularly toxic to the liver. Chronic exposure to glycol has been associated with encephalopathy and reproductive toxicity in laboratory animals.

296–298.   The answers are 296-a, 297-b, 298-g. *(LaDou, 2/e, pp 273, 320, 322, 329, 343, 519.)* Quartz is associated with silicosis, coal with the coal worker's pneumoconiosis, and cotton with byssinosis. Acrylic exposure may cause contact dermatitis and some respiratory and mucous membrane irritation.

299–300. The answers are 299-a, 300-c. *(LaDou, 2/e, pp 548, 554. Fauci, 14/e, pp 2532–2534.)* Parathion is an organophosphate pesticide. Pralidoxine can be given for the treatment of organophosphate (but not carbamate) poisoning. EDTA can be used as a chelating agent for lead. Amyl nitrite is used to treat cyanide poisoning, while flumazenil is used for benzodiazepine poisoning. Acetylcysteine is used for the treatment of acetaminophen poisoning.

301–303. The answers are 301-b, 302-c, 303-a. *(LaDou, 2/e, pp 222–223, 731.)* Although most occupational diseases are not infectious in origin, it is important to be aware of those that are. Packing and slaughterhouse employees, livestock producers, veterinarians, and hunters are at risk of developing brucellosis caused by a gram negative coccobacillus. Occupational infection usually results from inoculation through abraded skin or mucous membranes: gloves and goggles can prevent this form of spread. Infection can also result from ingestion of raw milk or animal tissues. *Legionella pneumophila* from contaminated aerosol can be disseminated in the ventilation systems through cooling towers, air-conditioning systems, humidifiers, and decorative fountains. Outbreaks can occur and air conditioner workers and others exposed can be at risk. Health care workers are at risk for hepatitis B and should be vaccinated. Farmers are at risk of developing fungal infections such as histoplasmosis and sporotrichosis.

304–305. The answers are 304-e, 305-f. *(LaDou, 2/e, p 244.)* Vinyl chloride and arsenic have been associated with liver cancer. Only vinyl chloride may be associated with brain cancer, but the data is weak. Bladder cancer can be caused by 4-aminobiphenyl, benzidine, coal tar and pitches, and β-naphtalamine. Lung cancer has been associated with many exposures: arsenic, asbestos, beryllium, cadmium, chromium, coal tar and pitches, mustard gas, nickel, radon, and vinyl chloride.

EPIDEMIOLOGY AND PREVENTION OF NONCOMMUNICABLE AND CHRONIC DISORDERS

Questions

DIRECTIONS: Each item below contains a question or an incomplete statement followed by suggested responses. Select the **one best** response to each question.

306. The American Academy of Pediatrics (AAP) revised its recommendations for fluoride supplements in 1995. What fluoride supplement would you recommend for a 4-year-old child if the water level in the community where she lives is 0.3 parts per million?

a. No supplement
b. 0.25 mg per day
c. 0.50 mg per day
d. 0.75 mg per day
e. 1.00 mg per day

Items 307–308

An asymptomatic 2-year-old child living in a delapidated older building in an inner-city neighborhood is screened for elevated lead levels. The results show a blood lead level of 30 μg/dL.

307. For which of the following conditions is this child at highest risk?

a. Decreased intelligence test scores
b. Impaired growth
c. High blood pressure
d. Chronic renal disease
e. Hepatic toxicity

308. Which intervention is the most important for this child?

a. Treatment with iron supplements
b. Chelation therapy with d-penicillamine
c. Chelation therapy with EDTA
d. Elimination of lead in the child's environment
e. Treatment with calcium supplements

309. A 25-year-old woman wants to lose weight before going on a trip to the Caribbean. She has joined a health club and signed up for classes with a stationary bike in which each 40-min session burns up 500 calories. She is taking two sessions a week. Assuming her caloric intake remains the same, how many weeks will it take to lose 6 pounds?

a. 5
b. 9
c. 15
d. 21
e. 27

Items 310–312

A 50-year-old man presents to a health center for routine care. His last visit was 5 years ago and he has no complaints. He has been smoking 1 pack of cigarettes a day since he was 15 years old. When counseled about his smoking, he says he has no intention of quitting and feels fine. He drinks two alcoholic beverages per week. Records show that his blood cholesterol is 235 mg/dL, with an HDL level of 40 mg/dL and an LDL level of 140 mg/dL. He has no family history of coronary artery disease (CAD). His height is 5'10" and he weighs 170 lbs. His blood pressure is 110/75 mm Hg.

310. What is the most appropriate approach to promote smoking cessation for this patient?

a. Refer him to classes for smoking cessation and reassess progress in 2 weeks
b. Provide self-help materials and reassess in 3 months
c. Prescribe nicotine replacement therapy and reassess progress in 2 weeks
d. Set a "quit date" with the patient and reassess his situation 2 days after this date
e. Give clear, personalized advice to quit and readdress the issue at the next visit

311. His blood cholesterol is repeated, and the results are the same. Which of the following is the most appropriate intervention for his lipid profile?

a. Repeat blood cholesterol in 1 year; no therapy is indicated
b. Recommend one alcoholic drink per day
c. Recommend dietary therapy
d. Recommend dietary and drug therapy
e. Recommend dietary therapy; if ineffective, add drug therapy

312. According to the U.S. Preventive Services Task Force, which additional preventive health measure is indicated?

a. Fecal occult blood testing (FOBT)
b. Influenza vaccine
c. Chest x-ray
d. Prostate-specific antigen (PSA)
e. Fasting blood glucose

313. Which of the following interventions is the most effective in the prevention and control of injuries?

a. Education
b. Economic incentives
c. Law enforcement
d. Engineering
e. Emergency response

314. Screening to detect problem drinking is recommended for all ages by the U.S. Preventive Services Task Force. The most effective method for early detection of alcohol abuse is

a. Liver function tests
b. Blood alcohol level
c. Questioning the family
d. Asking the patient about the quantity and frequency of alcohol use
e. Using a standardized questionnaire

315. A 16-year-old boy is diagnosed with depression following the divorce of his parents. He suffers from lack of appetite, insomnia, feelings of worthlessness, and difficulty in concentrating. He is given antidepressants and is referred to a psychologist for weekly psychotherapy visits. Which of the following is the most important risk factor for committing suicide?

a. Social isolation
b. Access to lethal medication
c. Noncompliance with antidepressant medication
d. Access to firearms
e. Alcohol abuse

316. The most important cause of years of potential life lost in the United States is

a. Cancer
b. Cardiovascular disease (CVD)
c. HIV infection
d. Injuries
e. Perinatal mortality

317. In most states, the legal limit for blood alcohol concentration allowed while operating a motor vehicle is

a. 10–20 mg/dL
b. 40–60 mg/dL
c. 80–100 mg/dL
d. 120–140 mg/dL
e. 150–200 mg/dL

318. An elderly homeless man in brought in by the police on a winter night because he was found wandering the streets confused and hallucinating. His consciousness is dulled and the ECG shows the following findings:

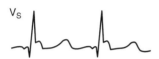

V_S

(Adapted, with permission, from Fauci AS, Braunwald E, Isselbacher KJ, eds., *Harrison's Principles of Internal Medicine*, 14th ed., New York, NY, McGraw-Hill, 1998: 1, 246.)

The most likely cause of these findings is

a. Hypothermia
b. Hypoglycemia
c. Acute alcohol intoxication
d. Dementia
e. Sepsis

319. A 27-year-old pregnant woman is brought to the emergency room with multiple ecchymoses to the chest and abdomen. Her breath smells of alcohol. The most likely cause of these findings is

a. Hepatic failure
b. Domestic violence
c. An accidental fall
d. An automobile accident
e. Disseminated intravascular coagulation

320. What proportion of the U.S. adult population is estimated to have a mental or emotional problem that requires therapy?

a. 1%
b. 5%
c. 15%
d. 25%
e. 40%

321. In country A, there are 35 new cases of breast cancer per 100,000 adult women per year. In country B, the number is 90 per 100,000. Which of the following is the most likely explanation?

a. Women in country A have a much higher rate of nursing their infants
b. Women in country A are less likely to smoke cigarettes
c. Women in country A receive more frequent preventive care, such as mammography
d. Treatment is much more successful in country A
e. Women in country A are younger

Items 322–323

The overall infant mortality rate (IMR) has declined in the United States since the beginning of the century. In some U.S. cities in 1900, up to 30% of infants would die before reaching the age of one. Overall rates have dropped from over 800 per 100,000 to less than 10 per 100,000 in 1998.

322. Which of the following is the main factor responsible for the decline in IMR during the 1990s?

a. Improvements in medical care
b. Reduction in sudden infant death syndrome
c. Reduction in vaccine-preventable diseases
d. Advances in prenatal diagnosis
e. Reduction in the incidence of low birth weight

323. Disparities in IMR persist among socioeconomic groups. Compared with white women, the IMR for African American women is

a. 25% higher
b. 50% higher
c. 100% higher
d. 50% lower
e. 75% lower

324. A 52-year-old woman presents to your office for her annual gynecological examination. She stopped menstruating about 6 months ago and is getting some hot flashes. Her history reveals that she drinks one glass of wine per day and smokes about 10 cigarettes per day. She does not exercise much and is overweight. Her most important risk factor for developing osteoporosis is

a. Smoking
b. Alcohol use
c. Lack of physical activity
d. Age
e. Obesity

325. A mother brings in her one-year-old child because she is concerned about potential exposure to lead. They have been making renovations in their older home and she is now considering moving to another house until the work is completed. You want to check the child's blood lead level. Which of the following is the most accurate method of screening for lead poisoning?

a. Erythrocyte protoporphyrin
b. Capillary blood lead
c. CBC
d. Venous blood lead
e. Ferritin

326. Which of the following types of cancer is the most frequent cause of gynecologic cancer deaths?

a. Ovarian
b. Cervical
c. Endometrial
d. Vaginal
e. Vulvar

327. You are employed by a government agency in the United States and are asked to make decisions about allocating funds for disease prevention. You consider the leading causes of death in the United States as guidance. In which order would you prioritize allocation of funds?

a. Heart disease, cancer, stroke, and chronic obstructive pulmonary disease (COPD)
b. Heart disease, cancer, COPD, and stroke
c. Heart disease, COPD, cancer, and stroke
d. Cancer, heart disease, COPD, and stroke
e. Accidents, COPD, heart disease, and stroke

Items 328–330

A 50-year-old woman comes for her periodical health examination. Her body mass index is 29 kg/m². Her blood pressure is 120/80. She has no family history of cardiovascular disease. Her total cholesterol is 200 mg/dL (5.2 mmol/L), her HDL is 35 mg/dL (0.9 mmol/L), and her LDL is 100 mg/dL (2.6 mmol/L).

328. This patient is at highest risk for developing which of the following conditions?

a. Stroke
b. Coronary artery disease
c. Non-insulin-dependent diabetes
d. Pulmonary embolism
e. Hypertension

329. This patient's weight increases the risk for which of the following cancers?

a. Breast, pancreas, and ovary
b. Endometrium, breast, and colon
c. Ovary, cervix, and colon
d. Cervix, ovary, and breast
e. Colon, endometrium, and ovary

330. The most appropriate initial intervention for weight loss is

a. Exercise
b. Surgery
c. Appetite-suppressive drugs
d. Diet with less than 25% of total calories from fat
e. Restriction to three meals per day

331. The effectiveness of the nicotine patch for smoking cessation increases with the intensity of the counseling provided. What percentage of smokers who use the patch and receive intensive counseling is still abstinent 6 months after the end of the treatment?

a.   10%
b.   25%
c.   40%
d.   55%
e.   70%

332. A mother brings her 14-year-old daughter to your office because she is concerned about her child's eating patterns. Her nutritional history reveals that she generally eats very little because she says she is not hungry. She occasionally engages in junk food binges with friends. She is often constipated. She exercises regularly. She is 5′6″ tall and weighs 108 pounds. Her menarche was at age 13. She stopped having periods 4 months ago. She says she has no concerns about her body image and thinks her mother is exaggerating because everyone in the family is tall and thin. The history and findings are most likely associated with

a.   Typical adolescent behavior
b.   Depression
c.   Hyperthyroidism
d.   Bulimia
e.   Anorexia

333. Which of the following is the most important risk factor for developing cervical cancer?

a.   Coitarche before age 18
b.   Herpes simplex virus infection
c.   Multiple sexual partners
d.   More than five years since the last Pap smear
e.   Human papillomavirus type 16

334. Above which level of desired body weight can someone be described as obese?

a.   110%
b.   120%
c.   130%
d.   140%
e.   150%

Items 335–336

In 1999, the CDC published the latest data for abortion surveillance (1996) in the United States. The abortion rate was 20/1000 women aged 15 to 44 years, the lowest since 1975. Mortality continues to be very low, with a case-fatality rate of less than 1/100,000 legal abortions. Monitoring abortion rates is useful for identifying women at high risk of unintended pregnancy and evaluating effectiveness of family-planning programs.

335. Among which age group is the highest abortion ratio?

a. <15 years
b. 15–19 years
c. 20–24 years
d. 35–39 years
e. >40 years

336. Approximately what percentage of abortions are performed before 13 weeks of gestation?

a. 25%
b. 50%
c. 60%
d. 80%
e. 90%

337. Which of the following patients is at highest risk for developing colon cancer?

a. A 50-year-old male with a long history of a diet high in animal fat
b. A 45-year-old female with irritable bowel syndrome
c. A 30-year-old with a history of familial polyposis
d. A 35-year-old male diagnosed with ulcerative colitis at age 25
e. A 45-year-old obese female with a diet low in fiber

338. The most frequent cause of death from unintentional injury in children under the age of 12 months is

a. Automobile accidents
b. Falls
c. Poisoning
d. Asphyxiation
e. Fire

339. The leading cause of death in males aged 25 to 44 in the United States is

a. Heart disease
b. Cancer
c. HIV infection
d. Homicide
e. Accidents

340. Which of the following 60-year-old patients is most likely to have an ischemic stroke within a year?

a. A male smoker
b. A male with hypertension
c. A male with an asymptomatic carotid bruit
d. A female with cardiovascular disease
e. A female with diabetes type 2

341. A 50-year-old alcoholic male presents to the emergency room with upper gastrointestinal (GI) bleeding. Examination reveals ataxia, confusion, and ophthalmoplegia. In addition to treating the GI bleeding, he would benefit from receiving which of the following?

a. Niacin
b. Pyridoxine
c. Folic acid
d. Thiamine
e. Cobalamin

342. In the 1990s, what proportion of adults in the United States was reported to be overweight?

a. <5%
b. 10–15%
c. 20–25%
d. 25–30%
e. 30–35%

343. You are asked to give a lecture on the epidemiology of cancer in the United States at your public health school alumni association. Which of the following statements best reflects the overall trends in the United States?

a. Incidence of cancer, as well as mortality rates, has been increasing in children
b. Incidence of lung cancer has been increasing in adults, but mortality rates have decreased
c. Incidence of cancer has remained stable in children, but mortality rates have decreased
d. Incidence of breast cancer in women has increased as well as mortality
e. Incidence of prostate cancer in men has increased as well as mortality

344. A 35-year-old woman presents to your office complaining of hair loss, bone pain, and dryness and fissures of the lips. She tells you that she has been taking large amount of vitamins in hopes of preventing cancer and infections. Her symptoms are most likely caused by an excess of

a. Vitamin A
b. Vitamin E
c. Vitamin C
d. Vitamin D
e. Vitamin K

Items 345–346

A 40-year-old man presents for his periodic health examination. He is overweight. His fasting blood sugar is 90 mg/dL, his total cholesterol is 210 mg/dL with a high-density lipoprotein (HDL) of 50 mg/dL and a low-density lipoprotein (LDL) of 130 mg/dL. His blood pressure is 120/80. He does not smoke. He has no cardiovascular or pulmonary symptoms. He admits to being a "couch potato" and not always eating healthily. You counsel him about increasing his physical activity and improving his diet.

345. For this patient, which of the following will most likely benefit from physical activity?

a. Blood pressure
b. Total cholesterol
c. HDL
d. LDL
e. Weight

346. Which of the following exercise regimens would be most appropriate to begin with?

a. Resistance training for 30 minutes 3 times a week
b. Jogging for 15 minutes 4 times a week
c. Brisk walking for 30 minutes 3 times a week
d. Jogging 60 minutes per day
e. Resistance training for 15 minutes every day

Items 347–349

You have just accepted a position as medical director for a large group practice and plan to develop guidelines for the provision of preventive services. You plan to use evidence-based medicine and follow the USPS Task Force recommendations. For each of the following interventions applied to the general population you will serve, choose the most appropriate group to screen.

347. Total cholesterol measurements

a. All men, women, and children
b. All men and women between the ages of 45 and 64
c. Only men between the ages of 35 and 64
d. Men between the ages of 35 and 64 and women between the ages of 45 and 64
e. All men and women, regardless of age

348. Blood pressure measurements

a. All men, women, and children
b. All men and women
c. Men and women starting at age 20
d. Men and women starting at age 30
e. Men and women starting at age 40

349. Mammography

a. Baseline at age 35, then yearly starting at age 40
b. Yearly starting at age 40
c. Yearly starting at age 50
d. Every three years starting at age 40
e. Every three years starting at age 50

Items 350–351

Breast cancer is the most frequent neoplasia among women. It is estimated that 1 woman out of every 8 will develop the disease over her lifetime.

350. What is the lifetime risk of developing breast cancer for a woman in whom the BRCA-1 has been detected?

a. 20%
b. 40%
c. 60%
d. 70%
e. 80% or more

351. Which of the following factors is most likely to decrease the lifetime risk of developing breast cancer in women?

a. Young age at menarche
b. Older age at menarche
c. Older age at menopause
d. Early menopause
e. Nulliparity

352. Which of the following mental disorders is more likely to occur in men compared to women?

a. Affective disorders
b. Anxiety disorders
c. Nonaffective psychosis
d. Substance abuse or dependence
e. Simple phobia

353. A 75-year-old widowed woman is brought to the emergency room because she fell while trying to go to the bathroom. Her daughter states that she has been getting more confused over the last few weeks. She has been disabled by arthritis for many years. She lives with her daughter who is single and works full-time. The examination reveals multiple ecchymoses on different areas of the body. She is very underweight, but her daughter states that she refuses to eat. Which of the following factors is most likely to cause the clinical findings?

a. Cancer
b. Abuse
c. Alzheimer's disease
d. Diabetes
e. Depression

354. Which of the following findings is the the most consistent among offenders in cases of child sexual abuse?

a. Alcohol abuse
b. Psychiatric illness
c. Stranger to the child
d. Prior sexual abuse
e. Relative or known to the child

Items 355–356

A 27-year-old man is brought to the emergency room by his friends because he has delusions about being followed by the FBI and has paranoid thoughts and behaviors.

355. Which of the following drugs is most likely to be causing this psychiatric presentation?

a. Cannabis
b. Heroin
c. LSD
d. Barbiturates
e. Cocaine

356. For what minimum length of time should this patient be enrolled in a drug treatment program for positive outcomes to occur?

a. 2 to 4 weeks
b. 1 to 3 months
c. 4 to 6 months
d. 6 to 12 months
e. 12 to 16 months

357. Which of the following factors is associated with decreased drug use among young adults?

a. Low socioeconomic status
b. Early drug use
c. Marriage
d. Parental drug use
e. Depression

358. You are employed by a state substance abuse program and are responsible for the design, implementation, and evaluation of drug prevention programs in schools. Which of the following attributes of the programs is most likely to impact drug use behavior?

a. Peer interaction
b. Length of program
c. Expert instruction
d. Size of the program
e. Socioeconomic status of students

359. A 20-year-old patient presents to the office for contraception counseling. Her history reveals no past medical problems. Her physical and pelvic examination is normal. She is sexually active with the same partner for 9 months. Which of the following contraceptive methods would be most appropriate?

a. Barrier method
b. Combined oral contraceptives
c. Progestin-only contraceptives
d. Intrauterine device (IUD)
e. Barrier method and combined oral contraceptives

360. A 30-year-old patient presents to your office for contraceptive counseling. She is divorced and has just started a new relationship. She wishes to use oral contraceptives because of their effectiveness. Her examination is normal. Which of the following factors would be considered a contraindication to their use?

a. Tobacco use
b. Vaginal bleeding
c. History of gestational hypertension
d. Polycystic breast disease
e. Migraines

361. The use of oral contraceptives will have the most impact on gynecological mortality by reducing the risk for which of the following cancers?

a. Ovarian
b. Breast
c. Cervical
d. Vulvar
e. Endometrial

362. Environmental tobacco smoke (ETS) is a major public health issue in the United States, particularly for children. Which of the following conditions is most affected by ETS?

a. Low birth weight
b. Middle ear infection
c. Bronchitis or pneumonia
d. Asthma
e. Lung cancer

363. A 28-year-old patient GoPoAo comes for her first prenatal visit at 6 weeks of pregnancy. Her examination is normal for gestational age. Her history reveals that she does not smoke. She drinks one glass of wine about two days a week. She has been married for three years and has only her husband as a sexual partner. She is employed as a paralegal. Her family history is negative. She is very concerned about preserving the mental and physical health of her baby. Which of the following interventions is most likely to reduce the risk of neurological defect in the infant?

a. Eliminating alcohol use
b. Folic acid supplements
c. Ultrasound
d. Amniocentesis
e. Alpha fetoprotein testing

364. A 57-year-old woman presents to the office because of vaginal bleeding. She had her menopause at age 50. She does not use hormonal replacement therapy. Her last periodic health examination was one year ago. The physical and pelvic examinations are nomal. Which of the following is the most likely diagnosis?

a. Atrophic vaginitis
b. Blood coagulation disorder
c. Endometrial carcinoma
d. Cervical carcinoma
e. Ovarian cancer

365. Which of the following groups of risk factors has been associated with endometrial cancer?

a. Hypertension, diabetes, and obesity
b. Family history, obesity, and nulliparity
c. Hypertension, oral contraceptives, and nulliparity
d. Family history, early pregnancy, and diabetes
e. Multiple pregnancies, obesity, and family history

366. A 50-year-old woman presents to the office complaining of abdominal pain and bloating. The pelvic examination reveals an adnexal mass of 5 cm. An ultrasound confirms the findings of a solid right ovarian mass of 7 cm. Ovarian cancer is suspected. Which of the following statements about the risk and screening for this disease is correct?

a. Routine screening for ovarian cancer with CA-125 is recommended
b. Screening with ultrasound is recommended
c. Family history is the most important risk factor for developing the disease
d. Oral contraceptives increase the risk of disease
e. Most patients are diagnosed early in the disease

Items 367–369

A 53-year-old woman presents to your office with questions about hormonal replacement therapy (HRT). She has been experiencing hot flashes and night sweats. She has not menstruated for one year. She has no risk factors for cardiovascular disease. She is 5′6″ and weighs 120 lbs. Her gynecological examination is normal as well as her Pap smear. Her breast examination and mammography are also normal. She wonders about the risks and benefits of HRT given her health status.

367. Which of the following lipid alterations are associated with menopause?

a. Decrease in total and HDL cholesterol
b. Increase in total and LDL cholesterol
c. Increase in HDL cholesterol, but no effect on total cholesterol
d. Increase in LDL cholesterol, but no effect on total cholesterol
e. No effect on HDL, LDL, or total cholesterol

368. HRT most increases her risk of developing which of the following conditions?

a. Hypertension
b. Thrombosis
c. Alzheimer's disease
d. Gallbladder disease
e. Endometrial cancer

369. The most benefit to be gained by HRT for this patient will be

a. Reduction of osteoporosis
b. Reduction of cardiovascular disease
c. Reduction of vasomotor symptoms
d. Reduction in the risk of breast cancer
e. Reduction in the risk of glucose intolerance

370. Which of the following is the leading cause of death for women of all ages in the United States?

a. Ischemic heart disease
b. Lung cancer
c. Breast cancer
d. Accidents
e. Stroke

371. For which of the following patients would aspirin chemoprophylaxis be CONTRAINDICATED?

a. An asymptomatic 52-year-old man at risk of CAD
b. An asymptomatic 60-year-old man with a prior myocardial infarction
c. A 55-year-old man with chronic stable angina
d. A 65-year-old man who has survived unstable angina and a myocardial infarction
e. A 45-year-old man with uncontrolled hypertension

372. Which of the following statements best reflects our current knowledge about prostate cancer?

a. African American men are at lower risk of developing the neoplasia
b. Prostate-specific antigen (PSA) is a sensitive screening tool
c. PSA is a specific screening tool
d. Digital rectal examination (DRE) can be helpful in detecting disease
e. Metastasis and an aggressive course is common

Items 373–374

The National Cholesterol Education Program has developed a two-step diet plan for persons with high cholesterol. Persons are considered at moderate risk of developing cardiovascular disease if their total cholesterol is between 200 and 239 mg/dL (5.2–6.2 mmol/L) and at high risk if their total cholesterol is 240 mg/dL or more (>6.2 mmol/L).

373. Which of the following dietary restrictions could be associated with a decrease in HDL?

a. Total dietary fat
b. Total dietary cholesterol
c. Total dietary carbohydrate
d. Total dietary polyunsaturated fat
e. Total dietary protein

374. After one of your patients fails to reduce her total blood cholesterol on the step one diet, you counsel her to start the step two diet. Which of the following modifications represent the main difference between the step one and the step two diet?

a. Dietary intake of total calories
b. Dietary intake of total carbohydrates
c. Dietary intake of saturated fat and cholesterol
d. Dietary intake of total protein
e. Dietary intake of total fat

375. Which of the following types of diets may reduce the risk of developing cancer?

a. Low-fiber diet
b. High-protein diet
c. High-fat diet
d. Diet rich in vitamin C and β-carotene
e. Diet rich in vitamin E

376. Which of the following statements best reflects the epidemiology of hypertension in the United States?

a. Systolic blood pressure tends to decrease with age
b. Alcohol and salt intake do not affect blood pressure
c. Family history is an important risk factor for developing hypertension
d. Obesity is not associated with hypertension
e. Only control of diastolic blood pressure has been shown to decrease mortality

377. Which of the following is the most important risk factor for developing insulin-dependent diabetes mellitus (IDDM)?

a. Country of residence
b. Male gender
c. Older age
d. Gestational diabetes in the mother
e. Presence of HLA-DR3

378. Which of the following complications is most likely to occur in a 35-year-old patient diagnosed with IDDM at age 15?

a. Retinopathy
b. Renal disease
c. Neuropathy
d. Stroke
e. Myocardial infarction

379. Which of the following diseases is the leading cause of end-stage renal disease (ESRD)?

a. Hypertension
b. Pyelonephritis
c. Diabetes
d. Glomerulonephritis
e. Obstructive nephropathy

380. Asthma is a common disease in children and the prevalence in the United States was estimated at 5% in 1992, a rise from 3% in 1982, with sharp declines noted from early childhood to adolescence. Which of the following factors is most strongly predictive of mortality due to asthma in children?

a. Age
b. Gender
c. Environmental pollutants
d. Overdependence on nebulizers
e. Severity of illness

381. A 52-year-old patient with chronic cough and shortness of breath is diagnosed with chronic obstructive lung disease. Which of the following factors is the most important contributor to this finding?

a. Tobacco use
b. Deficiency of α-antitrypsine
c. Asthma
d. Repeated childhood respiratory tract infections
e. Occupation

382. A 25-year-old woman presents to the delivery room in labor. She has had no prenatal care. The female newborn weighs 4.5 pounds and has episodes of seizures shortly after birth. Irritability and hypertonicity are also noted. The most likely cause for these findings in the newborn is

a. Cocaine use by mother
b. Alcohol consumption by mother
c. HIV in the mother
d. Syphilis in the mother
e. Heroin use by mother

383. Postmenopausal women who are not on hormone replacement therapy can benefit from daily calcium intake to reduce the risk of fractures secondary to osteoporosis. Which of the following is the recommended amount of calcium to be consumed daily?

a. 500 mg
b. 750 mg
c. 1000 mg
d. 1500 mg
e. 2000 mg

384. Consider the following skin lesion.

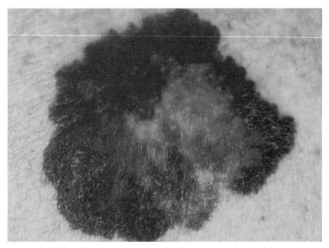

(Reproduced, with permission, from Fauci AS, Braunwald E, Isselbacher KJ, eds., *Harrison's Principles of Internal Medicine,* 14th ed., New York, McGraw-Hill, 1998.)

Which of the following statements best describes the epidemiology in the United States?

a. The incidence has been decreasing in recent years
b. Persons with fair complexions are at higher risk
c. Sunburn is not associated with the development of this lesion
d. Hereditary factors are not associated with this lesion
e. This lesion occurs primarily in children

385. A 22-year-old male presents to the student health center complaining of scrotal discomfort and swelling. He has no complaint of urethral discharge, fever, or genital lesions. He has been sexually active with the same partner for 3 years and uses condoms regularly as their method of birth control. He is otherwise healthy. The examination reveals a tender mass in the posterior aspect of the left testis. The most likely diagnosis is

a. Epididymitis
b. Lymphoma
c. Primary germ cell tumor
d. Varicoceles
e. Spermatoceles

386. Which of the following patients is at highest risk of adverse effects from iron deficiency anemia?

a. A postmenopausal woman
b. An elderly widow living alone
c. A breast-fed one-month-old infant
d. A 10-month-old with a diet of cow's milk
e. A 14-year-old with heavy periods

387. Which of the following public health interventions has been the most successful in preventing initiation of smoking or reducing the prevalence of smoking?

a. Media campaigns against smoking
b. Prohibiting the sale of tobacco to minors
c. Restrictions on indoor smoking
d. Lawsuits against the tobacco industry
e. Increases in cigarette prices through taxes

388. Which of the following statements most accurately describes depressive disorders?

a. They are associated with more frequent visits for physical symptoms
b. They mostly affect young married men
c. They are rarely encountered in ambulatory care
d. They can result in suicide in over 50% of cases
e. They are not a major economic burden in the United States

389. Public health efforts to prevent injuries have been particularly successful in reducing deaths from

a. Firearms
b. Fire
c. Motor vehicle accidents
d. Falls
e. Hypothermia

390. Biological basis for the occurrence of mental illnesses has been the subject of a number of studies. Schizophrenia has been linked with an increased activity of which of the following neurotransmitters?

a. Acetylcholine
b. Dopamine
c. Serotonin
d. GABA (gamma aminobutyric acid)
e. Norepinephrine

391. Which of the following acts as a cofactor in duodenal ulcer?

a. Cigarette smoking
b. Alcohol use
c. NSAID use
d. Blood group O
e. *Helicobacter pylori*

392. Consider the following population pyramid.

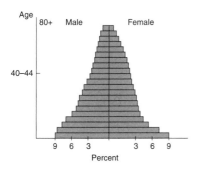

This pyramid is representative of which population structure?

a. Stationary
b. Expansive
c. Constrictive
d. Low fertility
e. High mortality

393. A 22-year-old female presents with a history of abdominal cramps, diarrhea, weight loss, and blood and mucus in the stools. Which of the following is a risk factor for developing this condition?

a. Oral contraceptives
b. Stress
c. Smoking
d. High-fat diet
e. Coffee

394. A 68-year-old man with controlled hypertension complains of gradual impairment of vision. His history further reveals that he was recently diagnosed with mild adult onset diabetes that is also well controlled. He is a retired fisherman. The most likely cause of his visual impairment is

a. Glaucoma
b. Cataract
c. Diabetic retinopathy
d. Macular degeneration
e. Xerophthalmia

395. A man afflicted with neurofibromatosis is the parent of a healthy, unafflicted female child. What is the probability that this child will transmit the disease to her own offspring if her partner is asymptomatic of the disease?

a. 25%
b. 50%
c. 100%
d. 0%
e. 75%

396. Which of the following genetic abnormalities is responsible for most cases of untreatable severe mental retardation?

a. Sex chromosome disorders
b. Autosomal chromosome disorders
c. X-linked recessive disorders
d. Autosomal dominant disorders
e. X-linked dominant disorders

397. Which of the following is the most cost-effective and safe public health measure today to prevent dental caries?

a. Water fluoridation
b. Proper nutrition
c. Regular dental visits
d. Promotion of regular flossing
e. Promotion of regular brushing

Items 398–401

Match each set of symptoms and signs with the dietary deficiency.

a. Vitamin A deficiency
b. Thiamine deficiency
c. Vitamin C deficiency
d. Vitamin D deficiency
e. Niacin deficiency
f. Vitamin E deficiency
g. Vitamin K deficiency

398. Petechiae, sore gums, hematuria, and bone or joint pain

399. Dermatitis, diarrhea, and delirium.

400. Edema, neuropathy, and myocardial failure.

401. Conjunctival xerosis, hyperkeratosis, and keratomalacia.

Items 402–404

Match the following behavior modification descriptions with the appropriate theoretical models.

a. Health belief model
b. Social learning theory
c. Theory of planned behavior
d. Theory of triadic influence
e. Stages of change theory

402. Precomtemplative, comtemplative, and ready for action.

403. Perceived susceptibility, severity, and benefits.

404. Outcome and efficacy expectations.

Items 405–408

For each description below, match the most appropriate level of prevention.

a. Primary prevention
b. Secondary prevention
c. Tertiary prevention
d. Primary and tertiary prevention
e. Primary and secondary prevention
f. Secondary and tertiary prevention

405. Treating a pregnant woman infected with syphilis.

406. Using condoms during sexual intercourse.

407. Pasteurizing milk.

408. Screening for hypertension.

Items 409–412

Match the effect of deficiency to the proper mineral.

a. Fluorine
b. Copper
c. Zinc
d. Sodium
e. Calcium

409. Poor mineralization of bones and teeth, osteoporosis.

410. Nausea, diarrhea, muscle cramps, dehydration.

411. Tendency to dental caries.

412. Dwarfism, hepatosplenomegaly, poor wound healing.

Items 413–415

Match the risk factor well documented for the type of cancer. Choose one or more than one.

a. Endometrial cancer
b. Cervical cancer
c. Breast cancer
d. Ovarian cancer
e. Colon cancer
f. Lung cancer
g. Prostate cancer
h. Esophageal cancer

413. Tobacco use.

414. Family history.

415. Alcohol.

Items 416–418

Match the ages with their leading causes of death.

a. Cancer
b. Heart disease
c. Suicide
d. Homicide
e. Injury
f. HIV/AIDS
g. Stroke

416. Ages 11 to 24.

417. Ages 25 to 64.

418. Age 65 and older

Items 419–422

Match the following populations to the disease which has a
higher prevalence.

a. Alpha-thalassemia
b. Beta-thalassemia
c. Cystic fibrosis
d. Hemophilia
e. Tay-Sachs disease
f. Sickle cell disease
g. Hemoglobin E

419. Southern Europe.

420. Africa.

421. Asia.

422. Ashkenazic Jews.

Items 423–424

Match the *typical use* failure rate
with the method of contraception.

a. Combined oral contraceptives
b. Intrauterine device (IUD)
c. Cervical cap
d. Diaphragm
e. Condoms
f. Spermicide
g. Withdrawal

423. 3%.

424. <1%.

EPIDEMIOLOGY AND PREVENTION OF NONCOMMUNICABLE AND CHRONIC DISORDERS

Answers

306. The answer is b. *(Wallace, 14/e, p 100.)* The decision to provide fluoride supplements (prescribed as drops or tablets) is based on the fluoride content of the drinking water and the age of the child. The latest recommendations from the AAP 1995 are as follows. No supplements are necessary before 6 months of age. If the water supply has levels less than 0.3 parts per million (ppm), the recommended dose is 0.25 mg/day for children aged 6 months to 3 years, 0.50 mg/day for children aged 3 to 6 years, and 1.00 mg/day for children aged 6 to 16 years. If the water level is between 0.3 and 0.6 ppm, supplement is not recommended for children younger than 3 years, 0.25 mg/day should be given to children aged 3 to 6 years, and 0.50 mg/day for children aged 6 to 16 years. No supplement is necessary if the level is 0.6 ppm or higher. Fluorosis, a white or brown discoloration of the teeth, can occur if ingestion of fluoride exceeds 4 to 8 mg/day.

307–308. The answers are 307-a, 308-d. *(Wallace, 14/e, p 1055. USPS Task Force, 2/e, pp 252–256.)* Even low lead levels can be detrimental to the intellectual performance of a child. The single most important intervention in reducing elevated blood lead levels in children is the elimination of lead in their environment, regardless of the level. Treatments should not be considered as substitutes for environmental interventions. Chelation therapy is recommended for all children with blood levels above 45 μg/dL. There is considerable debate about the use of chelation therapy when blood levels are between 20 and 45 μg/dL. The CDC recommends that an EDTA mobilization test be considered for children with blood levels between 25 and 44 μg/dL. If the test is positive, which, according to one study, can occur in up to 35% of children with venous lead levels between 25 and 35 μg/dL, then chelation therapy should be administered. Chelation agents include BAL, EDTA (edetate calcium disodium), DMSA, and d-penicillamine. Iron supplements are recommended if the child with elevated blood levels has iron deficiency anemia. Supplements also decrease the absorption of lead and may be considered even in the absence of iron deficiency.

309. The answer is d. *(Fauci, 14/e [full text], pp 456–458.)* It takes a 3500 deficit in calories to lose 1 pound of fat. If exercise only is used to produce the deficit of 1000 calories per week, it will take her 21 weeks to lose 6 pounds of fat. This will probably take her much longer than she thought. This is why dieting is often needed for weight-loss programs.

310–312. The answers are 310-e, 311-c, 312-a. *(Fauci, 14/e [full text], pp 2145–2146, 1350–1352. PARAN, J Resp Dis., 19:56–12, 1998. USPS Task Force, 2/e.)* For patients in a precontemplative stage of change, advising them to quit and personalizing the message to their risk factor is the best approach. It is important to continuously assess smoking status and advise to quit at every encounter to help motivate patients until they are ready for action. Those who are not ready to quit are unlikely to follow through on a quit date, go to smoking cessation classes, or use nicotine replacement therapy or self-help materials. According to the National Cholesterol Education Program (NCEP) guidelines, persons with borderline-high cholesterol 200 to 239 mg/dL with two or more risk factors for coronary heart disease (CHD), in this case, smoking and male = 45 years of age, should have a lipoprotein analysis performed, even if the HDL is 35 mg/dL. Dietary therapy would be the recommendation (no CHD, two or more risk factors) if the LDL is ≥130 mg/dL. Drug therapy is recommended by the NCEP if, despite dietary therapy, the following conditions are present: (1) LDL remains ≥190 mg/dL in the absence of CHD and fewer than two risk factors, (2) the LDL ≥160 mg/dL in the absence of CHD and two or more risk factors for CHD, (3) LDL ≥130 mg/dL in the presence of CHD. Dietary changes can reduce the cholesterol levels by as much as 15%, particularly if associated with weight loss and exercise. Screening for colon cancer is recommended for all persons age 50 and over. Fecal occult blood testing (FOBT) has been shown to be effective in reducing mortality from colon cancer by a randomized trial. Influenza vaccine is recommended for persons over the age of 65. None of the other measures are recommended for screening by the U.S. Preventive Services Task Force.

313. The answer is d. *(Wallace, 14/e, pp 1218–1219.)* Engineering methods have been the most effective to control injuries, particularly passive methods, such as automobile seatbelts and airbags. Education appears to be the least successful, in general, although it has resulted in behavioral change in some instances. The effectiveness of laws depends on their degree of enforcement. Emergency response will impact the damage resulting from injury, but not its prevention. It has less impact on morbidity than other methods.

314. The answer is e. *(USPS Task Force, 2/e, pp 567–582.)* The most effective method to detect early alcohol abuse is to use a structured questionnaire such as the CAGE or MAST. Abnormal serum gamma-glutamyltransferase (GGT) is neither sensitive nor specific enough to use for detection of early alcohol abuse. Blood alcohol levels are used to evaluate acute situations. Although asking the patient seems like a reasonable approach, reliability is variable. Finally, discussion with family members may be indicated if a problem is suspected.

315. The answer is d. *(Wallace, 14/e, pp 1043, 1250–1251.)* The proportion of firearms-related suicides has been increasing in recent years among youth and the elderly. Contrary to other methods, it is highly effective. The more difficult the access to a lethal method, the less likely someone will commit suicide. Limiting access to alcohol and drugs and compliance with therapy and medication will all be helpful to prevent a bad outcome. Social isolation contributes to a depressive state. Between 1955 and 1980, the rate of suicide among 15- to 24-year-olds tripled.

316. The answer is d. *(Wallace, 14/e, pp 163, 1212.)* Unintentional injury is the leading cause of death for all persons aged 1 to 24, making it the leading cause of years of potential life lost because of the young age of those most affected. Cardiovascular disease is still the overall leading cause of death in the United States, followed by cancer. HIV infection is the leading cause of death among persons aged 25 to 44.

317. The answer is c. *(Fauci, 14/e, p 2503.)* Behavioral, psychomotor, and cognitive changes can occur with blood alcohol levels of only 20 to 30 mg/dL. However, the legal limit of blood alcohol content (BAC) in *most* states is 80 to 100 mg/dL (0.1%), although there is a push toward lowering it further in some states. Levels of more than 300 to 400 mg/dL can be lethal. Ethanol either alone or with other intoxicants causes more toxic-overdose deaths than any other agent.

318. The answer is a. *(Fauci, 14/e [full text], pp 97, 1246; LaDou, 2/e, pp 139–141.)* Homelessness, alcohol use, and older age are all risk factors for developing *hypothermia,* which is defined as a core body temperature of 35° Celsius or less. Below 35° Celsius, consciousness is dulled and persons may be disoriented and confused. It is important to first take a core body temperature on this patient, preferably with a rectal thermocouple probe. The ECG shows the typical Osborn wave of hypothermia (a distinct convex "hump" at the J point).

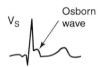

319. The answer is b. *(Wallace, 14/e, pp 854–855. Fauci, 14/e [full text], p 2503.)* It is estimated that between 20 and 25% of pregnant women suffer from domestic violence, and pregnancy is a particularly high-risk period for abuse. Battered women are much more likely to be injured on the chest, breasts, and abdomen than nonabused women. Over half of women who are battered eventually abuse alcohol.

320. The answer is c. *(Wallace, 14/e, p 1037.)* The estimated overall prevalence of mental disorders in the United States is 10 to 15% in children and 15% in adults. Anxiety disorders are the most prevalent, with an estimated 15 to 20% of clinic patients affected.

321. The answer is e. *(Fauci, 14/e [full text], p 562. Rosner, 5/e, p 594.)* The most important risk factor for breast cancer is age (as is often the case for most cancers): the rate in women 75 to 84 years old is about 50 times that of women 35 to 44 years old. If crude incidence rates are compared (new cases per 100,000 adult women), one country may have much larger numbers of women in the peak risk groups and have a much higher incidence for that reason. Therefore, either comparison of the age-specific rates for each age group or else some type of *age adjustment* is essential. Although nursing may have a protective effect on breast cancer, it is of nowhere near the magnitude of the effect of age. Cigarette smoke is not a major risk factor for breast cancer. Early diagnosis, if it had any effect, would be expected to increase the incidence rate since some cases might be discovered that otherwise might spontaneously resolve (or not be noticed before the woman died of another cause). Finally, efficacy of treatment might affect the death rate, but would not affect the incidence of the disease.

322–323. The answers are 322-a, 323-c. *(CDC, MMWR 48: 850–855, 1999. Schneider, pp 279–280.)* Improvements in medical care are largely responsible for the decreases in IMR. Sudden infant death syndrome (SIDS) has decreased by over 50% with the recommendations that babies be placed on their backs for sleeping. Although infant morbidity has decreased with better vaccine coverage, infant mortality has not been significantly affected. Advances in prenatal diagnosis have led in certain cases to early surgical interventions, thus reducing mortality due to congenital anomalies. Large racial differences still exist in infant mortality rates in the United States. The IMR for white women is 8 to 10 per 1000 live births, while that for African American women is 18 to 20 per 1000 live births.

324. The answer is d. *(Fauci, 14/e [full text], p 2248.)* Bone loss increases with age, particularly in women after menopause, when lack of estrogen accelerates the process. To a lesser extent, smoking, lack of physical activity, and alcohol abuse can also increase the risk of osteoporosis. Obesity, presumably because it is accompanied by an increase in estrogen production, does not increase the risk of osteoporosis.

325. The answer is d. *(USPS Task Force, 2/e, pp 251–252.)* Venipuncture is the best way to accurately measure blood lead levels. Capillary blood is often contaminated and results in falsely elevated levels. It is more cost-effective to collect venous blood initially than to do so only if the capillary blood level is high. Although many infants with lead poisoning will also have iron deficiency anemia, the complete blood count will not identify all cases of lead poisoning. The erythrocyte protoporphyrin is no longer recommended for screening as it will not identify lead levels below 25 µg/dL. It may be used for the detection of iron deficiency. Ferritin is used to estimate iron body stores.

326. The answer is a. *(Fauci, 14/e [full text], p 605.)* Over two-thirds of cases of ovarian cancer are detected when they are at an advanced stage. In

1996, there were 26,700 new cases diagnosed and 14,800 deaths. Ovarian cancer is responsible for 55% of all gynecologic cancers deaths, while endometrial and cervical cancers are responsible for 23 and 18%, respectively. Invasive cervical cancer is in theory 100% preventable because an effective screening test is available. A significant decrease has occurred in the last 45 years with the introduction of the Pap smear. Cancers of the vulva are less frequent, are more indolent, and account for only about 500 deaths annually. Vaginal cancer is rare.

327. The answer is a. *(USDHHS, Healthy People 2010, 1999.)* In 1997, heart disease was responsible for 31.4% of all deaths, cancer was responsible for 23.3%, stroke, 6.9%, chronic obstructive pulmonary disease (COPD), 4.7%, and unintentional injuries, 4.1%.

328–330. The answers are 328-c, 329-b, 330-d. *(Fauci, 14/e, pp 459, 466.)* Type 2 diabetes mellitus is almost nonexistent in individuals with a BMI below 22kg/m². Prevention of obesity prevents diabetes. Even modest weight reduction (5 to 10 kg) decreases insulin resistance and the resulting hyperinsulinemia. Increased mortality from obesity results from cardiovascular disease, hypertension, diabetes, and some types of cancer. Obesity is associated with hypertriglyceridemia, decreased HDL, and increased LDL. Obesity is a risk factor particularly for endometrial cancer, although it may also increase the risk of postmenopausal breast cancer and colon cancer. Diet is the first step in reducing weight. Reducing or eliminating alcohol intake and taking frequent small meals helps to reduce food intake. Exercise helps maintains weight loss, but is not a primary strategy. Medication is reserved for women with a BMI above 30 or 27 kg/m² if comorbidity is present, and surgery for above 35 kg/m².

331. The answer is b. *(AHCPR, 1996. Wallace, 14/e, p 830.)* A meta-analysis of all studies evaluating transdermal nicotine therapy reveals that with high-intensity counseling, "quit" rates at the end of treatment and after 6 months are 41.6 and 26.5%, respectively. With low-intensity counseling, the quit rate is 22.8% at the end of treatment and 19.5% after 6 months. Overall, there is a 21.8% abstinence rate after 6 months for all patch studies, compared with 9.4% with placebo. Nicotine replacement therapy (multiple modalities are now available) or Bupropion should be offered, unless contraindicated, to all smokers who are ready to quit.

332. The answer is e. *(Fauci, 14/e [full text], p 463.)* Anorexia occurs predominantly in females and begins either before or shortly after puberty. Binge eating may occur, although it is uncommon and more closely associated with bulimia. Weight is decreased in anorexia whereas it is near normal in bulimia. Ritualized exercise is usual in anorexia, but not in bulimia. Amenorrhea is always present in anorexia because of weight loss. Antisocial behavior is more frequently associated with bulimia than with anorexia, and the depression in bulimia tends to be more severe than in anorexia, making suicide a definite risk.

333. The answer is e. *(Fauci, 14/e [full text], p 609.)* HPV DNA is present in 95% of all cervical cancers and is the most important risk factor, in fact, etiologic agent, for developing neoplasia. Only certain types of HPV have oncogenic potential: 16, 18, 31, 45, and 51–53. Most patients who die from invasive cervical cancer have never had a Pap smear in their lives. Early initial sexual activity, presumably because the cervix is more susceptible to agents which might induce cancer, and multiple sexual partners are also risk factors. Smoking increases the risk of developing neoplasia.

334. The answer is c. *(Fauci, 14/e [full text], pp 454–456.)* Although a percentage of ideal body weight can be used, obesity is best defined by measuring the body mass index: (weight in kg/height in m²) > 26 BMI. Fat mass can also be a useful measure: obesity is arbitrarily considered to be present when body fat is >25% in men and >30% in women.

335–336. The answers are 335-a, 336-e. *(CDC, MMWR 48[SS-5], 1999.)* *Abortion ratio* refers to the number of abortions per 100 live births, while the *abortion rate* refers to the number of abortions per 1000 women 15 to 44 years of age. Abortion rates increased from 1970 to 1978, remained relatively stable until 1990, when they began declining. Abortion ratios tend to be higher at the extremes of reproductive age (<15 and >40 years). The great majority of abortions are performed at less than 12 weeks of gestation. The percentage of women who obtained late abortions are highest among women less than age 15.

337. The answer is c. *(Fauci, 14/e [full text], pp 572–573.)* As much as 25% of patients with colorectal cancer have a family history of the disease. Offsprings of persons with familial polyposis have a 50% probability of developing the disease, and annual flexible colonoscopy is recommended until age

35. It will usually be identified by age 25. Almost all patients who are not treated for these colonic polyps will develop cancer by age 40. There has been an association described between diets high in animal fat and colon cancer, but the data is less convincing for high-fiber diets decreasing the risk. The risk of developing colon cancer in patients with inflammatory bowel disease ranges from 8 to 30% after 25 years of the disease. Irritable bowel syndrome is not a risk factor for developing colon cancer. Obesity can also increase the risk of colon cancer, but to a lesser degree than the other factors.

338. The answer is d. *(Wallace, 14/e, pp 1212–1213. USPS Task Force, 2/e, pp 661–664.)* Injuries are the leading cause of death in the younger members of the U.S. population. Asphyxiation occurs mainly in older adults age 75 and over and young children age 4 and younger. In 1991, fires and burns were the second leading cause of death resulting from unintentional injuries in children 9 and younger. Falls are a common cause of injury in children under the age of 5, but they rarely result in death. Drowning occurs mainly in older children.

339. The answer is c. *(Wallace, 14/e, p 1229. USPS Task Force, 2/e, p 303.)* The leading cause of death for men between the ages of 25 and 44 is now HIV infection, followed by unintentional injuries, heart disease, cancer, and homicide. Homicide is the leading cause of death for African American men between the ages of 15 and 24.

340. The answer is b. *(Wallace, 14/e, p 102. Fauci, 14/e [full text], pp 1384, 2336.)* Hypertension is a major risk factor for hemorrhagic (through elevated arterial pressure and microaneurysm) and ischemic stroke. Treatment of high blood pressure is the most efficacious way to prevent stroke, including in the elderly. Other risk factors for strokes include smoking, vascular disease, and diabetes mellitus. In individuals with cerebral vascular disease, the risk of developing a stroke within one year for a patient with an asymptomatic carotid disease is 1.3% and with a transient ischemic attack is 3.5%; the greatest risk is for the patient with ≥70% symptomatic carotid stenosis (15%).

341. The answer is d. *(Fauci, 14/e [full text], pp 145, 483–484, 656–657.)* The patient has Charcot's triad of ataxia, confusion, and ophthalmoplegia, which occurs in malnourished individuals. Parenteral thiamine may reverse the disease if given within a few days of the occurrence of symptoms. Prolonged untreated deficiencies can result in permanent damage.

Vitamin B_{12} (cobalamin) deficiency, which can occur in pernicious anemia, causes a spinal cord syndrome resulting in sensory loss with depressed tendon reflexes. Niacin deficiency results in pellagra and is associated with a high uptake of maize in the American South. Pyridoxine or vitamin B_6 deficiency is associated with the intake of certain drugs, such as izoniazid, and results in abnormal tryptophan metabolism and convulsions. Folate deficiency can result in glossitis, cheilosis, and diarrhea, but does not cause neurological problems (except for neural tube defects during pregnancy).

342. The answer is e. *(Fauci, 14/e [full text], p 456.)* Data from the National Center for Health Statistics show the rise in prevalence of obesity from 26% in 1960–1962 to 35% in 1988–1991. This rise has been more important in the last 10 years (was 27% in 1976–1980).

343. The answer is c. *(Wallace, 14/e, pp 911–912.)* Reductions of mortality in cancer in children result from prolonged survival due to improved therapy. The incidence of breast cancer and prostate cancer has increased probably largely due to increased screening; however, mortality rates have remained rather stable, reflecting little improvement in survival. There has been both an increase in lung cancer rates (due to smoking) as well as mortality.

344. The answer is a. *(Fauci, 14/e [full text], p 487.)* Chronic toxicity of vitamin A (25,000 units or more for a protracted period) symptoms include bone pain, hyperostosis, hair loss, dryness and fissures of the lips, and weight loss. High doses of vitamin C for long periods can cause an increase in the risk of oxalate kidney stones and cause uricosuria. Vitamin E excess is present in persons receiving anticoagulants and in premature infants and can prolong prothrombin time. Vitamin D excess will result in hypercalcemia. Vitamin B_1 or thiamine excess has not been described. Vitamin K excess will result in blocking the effect of anticoagulants. Excess most frequently occurs in fat-soluble vitamins (A, D, K, E).

345–346. The answers are 345-e, 346-c. *(Fauci, 14/e, p 47. USPS Task Force, 2/e, pp 612–619. USDHHS, Healthy People 2010, 1999.)* The patient's blood pressure and glucose are normal. His HDL is more than 35. However, his obesity puts him at risk of developing hypertension, type 2 diabetes, and CVD. An exercise program, in addition to diet, would help him lose weight. Physical activity may decrease the risk of coronary artery disease by as much as 35%. HDL has been shown to increase in men following a rigorous training program. The optimal cardiovascular protection can be achieved by doing 20 to 30 minutes of vigorous activity three or more times per week. However, exercise should be approached gradually as a sudden onset may precipitate myocardial infarction. Successful programs should be integrated into everyday life activities.

347–349. The answers are 347-d, 348-a, 349-c. *(USPS Task Force, 2/e, pp 29–30, 46–47, 83–84.)* The USPS Task Force recommends that blood pressure be taken routinely at all ages. Cholesterol is recommended only in adults, unless there is a family history of very high cholesterol or premature coronary heart disease. Mammography is recommended for women over the age of 50: the issue of mammography in women between the ages of 40 and 50 is controversial, and recommendations for or against cannot be made. Some professional organizations such as the American Cancer Society (ACS) recommend screening in women starting at age 40, while others recommend that individual decisions be made. Any decrease in mortality in this age group will be less than for those over 50.

350–351. The answers are 350-e, 351-b. *(Fauci, 14/e [full text], pp 562–563. USPS Task Force, 2/e, p 74.)* Having the BRCA-1 gene is associated with a very high risk of developing breast cancer, with a 70% chance before age 60. Late menarche and early menopause (less lifetime exposure to estrogen) can reduce the risk of developing breast cancer by 50 to 60% and 35%, respectively. Full-term pregnancy before age 18 can decrease the risk by 30 to 40%. Nulliparity is a risk factor for the disease.

352. The answer is d. *(Wallace, 14/e, p 1040.)* Overall, women are more likely to suffer from affective disorders (depressive and manic) and anxiety disorders (phobia and anxiety). Prevalence of any substance abuse/dependence is 16.6% in men and 6.6% in women.

353. The answer is b. *(Wallace, 14/e, pp 1247–1249.)* Elders who are disabled are more likely to suffer from physical abuse or neglect. Most abuse is by a relative, and most abused elders are likely to live with the abuser, who is often stressed both emotionally and financially as the elder requires more care. Many abused elders become depressed as a result of abuse.

354. The answer is e. *(Wallace, 14/e, pp 1244–1245.)* Most offenders are males, which clearly distinguishes sexual abuse from other forms of abuse or neglect. They are predominantly either a relative of the child (father, uncle, older brother) or a nonrelative known to the child. Abuse by a stranger is far less frequent. Some studies have found that up to 33% of offenders have been victims of sexual abuse themselves. The use of alcohol is often related to the act. Difficulties with adult heterosexual relationships, problems with capacity for behavioral inhibition, and deviant sexual arousal patterns have all been described, but not specific psychiatric illnesses.

355–356. The answers are 355-e, 356-d. *(Wallace, 14/e, pp 864–874. Fauci, 14/e [full text], p 2513.)* Chronic cocaine use can occasionally cause paranoid behavior. Hallucinations and acute psychosis with extreme violent behavior is associated with LSD. Chronic use of LSD may lead to similarities with mentally ill persons reporting profound religious experiences. Chronic use of marijuana can lead to disinterest in desirable social goals. Major issues about chronic opiate intake is related to acquiring HIV and other infectious diseases. According to the Treatment Outcome Prospective Study, the most important predictor of success of drug treatment was length of time in the program, regardless of type of drugs used. Being in a program for at least 6 to 12 months was associated with abstinence, reduction of crime, and full-time employment.

357. The answer is c. *(Wallace, 14/e, p 870.)* Older age at initiation of drug use, employment, and marriage are factors associated with decreased drug use in young adults. Parental drug use and educational level, peer drug use, early drug use, sensation seeking, deviance, poor school grades, depression, agression, and low socioeconomic status are all risk factors associated with drug use.

358. The answer is a. *(Wallace, 14/e, pp 870–871.)* The single most important factor that has had some impact on the ultimate outcome, that is, drug use, is interaction with peers, regardless of socioeconomic status or race/ethnicity. Larger programs have been less effective than smaller programs in reducing drug use regardless of type.

359. The answer is e. *(Fauci, 14/e [full text], p 2111. Wallace, 14/e, pp 1189–1192.)* Only barrier methods, particularly condom use, can reduce the risk of acquiring sexually transmitted diseases (STDs). However, their ability to reduce the rate of pregnancy is less than combined oral contraceptives (COC). Progestin-only pills are slightly less effective than COC. The IUD is not recommended for young women: they may be at higher risk of STDs, which may increase the risk of PID and infertility.

360. The answer is b. *(Fauci, 14/e [full text], p 2112. Wallace, 14/e, pp 1189–1192.)* Abnormal vaginal bleeding needs to be investigated before oral contraceptives can be used. Migraine headaches are not a contraindication to their use: some patients experienced improvement in the headaches. A trial can be done with a low dose. Gestational hypertension is not a contraindication to OCs: blood pressure can be monitored after administration of a low-dose OC. Tobacco use would be an absolute contraindication if the patient was 35 or older. History of stroke, thrombophlebitis, pulmonary embolism, and coronary artery disease are all absolute contraindications to OCs.

361. The answer is a. *(USPS Task Force, 2/e, pp 756–758.)* Oral contraceptives have been shown to reduce the risk of ovarian cancer, the leading cause of death from gynecological cancer, by up to 80%. They can also reduce the risk of endometrial cancer. They have no effect on the risk of developing vulvar cancer. The issue of whether they increase the risk of breast cancer and cervical cancer is debatable. Any potential increase in the risk of breast cancer is likely to be very small and to occur only in a certain subgroup of women: the benefits of using OCs far outweigh any risks.

362. The answer is d. *(Medical Foundation report, 1999.)* Estimated annual morbidity in nonsmokers exposed to ETS is 400,000 to 1 million children affected by exacerbation of their asthma; 8000 to 26,000 children affected by asthma induction; 700,000 to 1.6 million physician office visits for middle ear infections; 150,000 to 300,000 cases of bronchitis or pneumonia in infants less than 18 months old; and 9700 to 18,600 cases of low birth weight. Lung cancer is an adult disease: an estimated 3000 deaths can be attributed to exposure to ETS.

363. The answer is b. *(Wallace, 14/e, p 1054. USPS Task Force, 2/e, pp 568–569.)* Folic acid use during the first trimester of pregnancy has been shown to decrease the incidence of neural tube defect, which is often associated with hydrocephalia, which in turn may be associated with intellectual disability that can be severe. In fact, folic acid supplements are recommended beginning one month prior to conception, so for all women capable of becoming pregnant. It is advisable to counsel women to avoid alcohol during pregnancy, although the risk of fetal alcohol syndrome is increased with 14 drinks per week or more. The effect of lower levels of drinking has been inconsistent.

364. The answer is c. *(Fauci, 14/e [full text], pp 608–609.)* Endometrial cancer most often presents with vaginal bleeding (80%) and is the most common postmenopausal gynecological cancer. Atrophic vaginitis does not present as spontaneous vaginal bleeding. A blood coagulation disorder would most likely present with other signs (petechia, bleeding gums) and symptoms. An endometrial biopsy should be performed in this situation.

365. The answer is a. *(Fauci, 14/e [full text], pp 605–606, 609, 2112.)* Hypertension, diabetes, low fertility, obesity, and late menopause have all been associated with endometrial cancer. Family history is not a risk factor. The use of oral contraceptives has been shown to decrease the risk.

366. The answer is c. *(Fauci, 14/e [full text], p 606. USPS Task Force, 2/e, pp 161–184.)* Family history is a major risk factor for the disease. Most patients are diagnosed when the cancer has spread beyond the true pelvis. Earlier detection of the disease could improve survival, but the performance of tests has been disappointing. Half of the women with stage I and II ovarian cancer have CA-125 levels of less than 65 U/ml, while elevated levels are associated with nonmalignant disorders. Studies have shown that routine ultrasound has a low yield in detecting cancer and generates a large amount of false-positives. Routine screening, either with ultrasound or CA-125, is not recommended.

367–369. The answers are 367-b, 368-e, 369-a. *(USPS Task Force, 2/e, pp 829–838. Fauci, 14/e [full text], p 2113 (Nawaz, AJPM 17:250–254, 1999.)* Menopause is associated with substantial rises in total and LDL cholesterol. Some studies have suggested that HRT appears to decrease the incidence of Alzheimer's disease. HRT has no effect on gallbladder disease and hypertension. Unopposed estrogen therapy particularly increases the risk of endometrial cancer. Adding progesterone to the regimen significantly reduces this risk, but does not eliminate it. Thin, white women are particularly at risk of osteoporosis. Although there is definitely a benefit from reduction of CVD, this patient has little risk factors for developing the disease and may benefit more from the reduction of fractures. HRT may increase the risk of developing breast cancer and may slightly increase the risk of deep venous thrombosis (DVT). On a population basis, the benefits of HRT (reduction in cardiovascular diseases and osteoporosis) are of greater magnitude than the risks (DVT, endometrial and breast cancer). On an individual basis, risks and benefits should be assessed based on risk profile.

370. The answer is a. *(Fauci, 14/e [full text], p 21.)* Heart disease remains the leading cause of death among women of all ages, followed by cerebrovascular disease, lung cancer, and breast cancer. Breast cancer is the leading cause of death for women between the ages of 45 and 54. Motor vehicle accidents are the leading cause of death for women aged 24 to 34.

371. The answer is e. *(Fauci, 14/e [full text], pp 747, 1372. USPS Task Force, 2/e, pp 849–850.)* This patient is at high risk of a hemorrhagic stroke. Aspirin can reduce the risk of thrombotic stroke. Other contraindications for aspirin use include gastrointestinal bleeding, allergy, diabetic retinopathy, kidney and liver disease, and dyspepsia. There is currently no data that aspirin prophylaxis is as effective in women.

372. The answer is d. *(Fauci, 14/e [full text], pp 598–602.)* Prostate cancer is the most common malignancy in men, is rare before the age of 50, and its incidence increases with age. African American men are at higher risk of the disease. PSA is elevated in only 65% of cases of prostate cancer and it lacks specificity because it can also be elevated in benign prostatic hyperplasia, prostatitis, and prostatic infarction. For this reason, it is not recommended for routine screening by the USPS Task Force, in addition to the fact that it is not clear whether screening improves survival. Treatment also leads to serious complications that may impact quality of life. Although its value for routine screening has not been established, some professional organizations, such as the American Cancer Society, recommend PSA screening for all men over the age of 50 in addition to DRE. A PSA of 4 ng/ml or less is considered normal. A PSA >10 ng/ml would be indicative of cancer, regardless of the results of DRE. How to manage the patient with a negative DRE and a PSA between 4 and 10 ng/ml is unclear. Refinements of the use of PSA in association with other measures (such as prostate volume, rate of rise, age of patient, etc.) are under investigation. Indolent, slow growth is frequent in prostate cancer.

373–374. The answers are 373-a, 374-c. *(Fauci, 14/e [full text], pp 466–467.)* Both step 1 and 2 recommend that total dietary fat represents <30% of kcal intake, carbohydrate, 50–60%, protein, 10–20%, monosaturated fat and polyunsaturated fat represent 10–15% and <10% of kcal intake, respectively. Step one recommends that total cholesterol intake be less than 300 mg/dL, while step two recommends less than 200 mg/dL. The other difference is in the intake of saturated fat: 8–10% of total kcal for step one versus <7% for step two. Reducing the total fat intake has been associated with a decrease in HDL and an increase in triglycerides in some patients (potentially due to the increase in carbohydrate and polyunsaturated fats). They should be advised to substitute monosaturated fat (which increases HDL and decreases LDL) for saturated fat.

375. The answer is d. *(Fauci, 14/e [full text], p 467.)* A diet rich in fiber with plenty of vegetables and fruits, particularly those rich in β-carotene and vitamin C, and low in fat (30% or less in total kcal intake) may reduce the risk of developing cancer. Limiting or eliminating alcohol, avoiding obesity, and limiting the consumption of cured or smoked meats may also be helpful.

376. The answer is c. *(Wallace, 14/e, pp 950–953.)* Alcohol use has been shown to increase blood pressure. There is a favorable association between low salt intake and change in blood pressure with age. Systolic blood pressure tends to increase with age. Both systolic and diastolic blood pressure have independent contributions to the risk of mortality. Obesity is associated with hypertension.

377. The answer is e. *(Wallace, 14/e, pp 971–972.)* There are large differences in the incidence of IDDM between countries: with Finland having the largest incidence (30/100,000) and Mexico having the lowest (less than 0.5/100,000). The incidence in the United States is 15/100,000 and has remained stable over the last 30 years. Rates are similar between males and females. Incidence peaks at adolescence, and then drops dramatically. The incidence decreases over the summer months, suggesting a link with viral infections. There is strong association between IDDM and the HLA region of chromosome 6. Approximately 95% of all IDDM patients are HLA-DR3, HLA-DR4, or both.

378. The answer is a. *(Wallace, 14/e, pp 974–975.)* After 20 years of IDDM, virtually all patients have some form of diabetic retinopathy. As many as 70% may also have proliferative changes that may lead to blindness. About 40% of patients with IDDM eventually develop significant proteinuria and renal disease. Lower blood sugar levels can prevent or delay clinical neuropathy which can occur in as much as 70% of patients after 30 years. CVD increases with years of duration and is the leading cause of mortality in patients with IDDM for over 30 years.

379. The answer is c. *(Wallace, 14/e, p 965.)* From 1989 to 1993, in the United States, diabetic nephropathy accounted for 37.5% of all ESRD, followed by hypertensive nephropathy (30.3%), glomerulonephritis (12.3%), cystic kidney disease (3%), interstitial nephritis (3%), collagen vascular disease (2.2%), and obstructive nephropathy (2%).

380. The answer is e. *(Wallace, 14/e, p 985.)* Risk factors for developing asthma include male gender, family history, respiratory tract infection, ambient air pollution, environmental tobacco smoke, and bronchial hyperactivity. Age-adjusted mortality from asthma has increased in the United States, although it is still a rare event. It is more common among adults than children. Studies have demonstrated that the severity of illness is the most important predictor of death. Recently, discontinuation of inhaled steroids has been proven to be a risk factor for asthma-related death.

381. The answer is a. *(Fauci, 14/e [full text], p 1452. Wallace, 14/e, p 986.)* From 80 to 90% of all cases of COPD in the United States is attributable to cigarette smoking. Some occupations with particle or dust exposure may also be associated with COPD. Deficiency of α-antitrypsine is uncommon and is generally associated with emphysema. There is some data to suggest that severe viral pneumonia early in life may lead to obstructive disease.

382. The answer is a. *(Wallace, 14/e, p 1055. USPS Task Force, 2/e, p 585.)* The findings are typical of cocaine use during pregnancy, which has also been associated with impaired fetal growth and increased risk of placenta abruptio. Infants exposed to opiates during pregnancy may exhibit symptoms of withdrawal. Fetal alcohol syndrome is characterized by microcephaly, stunting, flattened nasolabial facies, and narrow palpebral tissues. Congenital syphilis had been described in Chapter 2. HIV infection is asymptomatic at birth.

383. The answer is d. *(Fauci, 14/e [full text], p 2252. USPS Task Force, 2/e, p 634.)* Calcium intake in early childhood and adolescence can increase bone mineral density in women. It may also decrease bone loss at later years. Adolescents should take 1200–1500 mg/day and women 25 to 50 years of age should take 1000 mg/day. Postmenopausal women will probably benefit more from HRT to reduce osteoporosis, but calcium supplements of 1000–1500 mg/day may also be helpful. For those without HRT, a dose of 1500 mg/day is recommended.

384. The answer is b. *(Fauci, 14/e [full text], pp 541–542.)* The incidence of melanoma, which occurs primarily in adults, but could occur in teens, is on the rise in the United States. Sunburn has been associated with the development of the lesion. Other risk factors include a family history, the presence of a clinically atypical mole, a giant congenital melanocytic nevus, and the presence of a higher-than-average number of ordinary melanocytic nevi (>50; ≥2 mm) and immunosuppression.

385. The answer is c. *(Fauci, 14/e [full text], p 602.)* Epididymitis is unlikely in this patient given the sexual history, as well as the physical examination. Lymphoma occurs primarily in men over the age of 50. History and physical examination rule out orchitis (painful testis but no mass), varicoceles ("bag of worms"), and spermatoceles (painless mass). Patients may often present with these symptoms instead of the pathognomonic painless testicular mass. Primary germ cell tumors account for 95% of all testicular cancers. Cure rates are 90% for noninvasive tumors, and with the advent of cisplastin chemotherapy, cure rates of 70 to 80% are expected for metastatic cancers. Most tumors occur in men between the ages of 20 and 40. Cryptorchidism is a risk factor for the disease. Orchiopexy can reduce this risk.

386. The answer is d. *(USPS Task Force, 2/e, pp 239–241.)* Infants on cow's milk are at highest risk of iron deficiency anemia, which can be associated with abnormal growth and development. A study on iron therapy in a high-risk population has shown an important effect of iron therapy on development. Postmenopausal women are not at high risk of anemia. Elderly persons, because of poor diet, may be at higher risk. Breast feeding (with iron-fortified supplements added at 4 to 6 months) and feeding iron-fortified formula can reduce the incidence of iron deficiency anemia.

387. The answer is e. *(Schneider, pp 227–236.)* Studies have shown that teenagers are very sensitive to the price of cigarettes. Some studies have shown that an increase in the price of cigarettes by 10% can reduce the number of teens who smoke by 7 to 12%. Inversely, when the price of a brand of cigarettes particularly favored by teens was reduced by the tobacco company, the proportion of teens who smoked increased from 23.5 to 28% over three years.

388. The answer is a. (*USPS Task Force, 2/e, p 541. Fauci, 14/e [full text], pp 2491–2492.*) Depression is more common in persons who are young, female, divorced, single, separated, seriously ill, or have a prior history or family history of depression. Suicide occurs in 15% of untreated major depressive disorders, with most patients having sought help from a physician within the month. Depressed patients frequently present with a variety of physical complaints, often leading to unnecessary procedures and intervention. The annual economic burden has been estimated to be almost $44 billion.

389. The answer is c. (*Christoffel, pp 131, 147–148.*) Improved motor vehicle and highway design, increased use of safety belts and motorcycle helmets, and enforcement of laws regarding drinking and driving and speeding have saved 240,000 lives between 1966 and 1990, making this one of the most successful injury prevention programs. Similar results can be possible with other types of injury, which in fact could almost all be preventable, by using a public health approach. Physicians can play an important part by counseling their patients about injury prevention, a cornerstone of pediatric practice (anticipatory guidance).

390. The answer is b. (*Fauci, 14/e [full text], pp 2487, 2488, 2493, 2500.*) Panic disorders appear to be associated with increased noradrenergic discharges, general anxiety disorders with aberrations of benzodiazepine GABA receptors, and depression associated with lower levels of serotonin. Of additional interest: risk factors for schizophrenia include genetic vulnerability (i.e., family history), early developmental insults, and winter birth.

391. The answer is e. (*Wallace, 14/e, pp 992–994.*) Eradication of H. pylori heals ulcers except for those caused by NSAID. *H. pylori* is not a *cofactor* when NSAID use is the etiologic factor. Cigarette smoking (RR = 2), use of NSAID in persons over age 55 (RR = 2–6), family history (RR = 3), gastric hyperacidity (RR = 7), and blood group O (RR = 1.3) are all *risk factors* for duodenal ulcers. No independent association with alcohol use has been established.

392. The answer is b. *(Wallace, 14/e, pp 48–53.)* High-fertility populations have pyramids where the base is wider than the middle and the top. There are three basic patterns of interaction of population structure, fertility, and mortality: expansive with a high proportion of children; stable, where there is a moderate proportion of children and zero growth (fertility and mortality is constant); and constrictive, where the proportion of children is insufficient to maintain growth. Fertility affects the pattern more than mortality.

393. The answer is a. *(Wallace, 14/e, pp 997–999.)* The use of oral contraceptives has been linked to increased risk of developing ulcerative colitis (UC). Smoking actually decreases the risk (although no one would advocate smoking to decrease the risk . . .). Diet, coffee consumption, and stress have not been shown to be risk factors. The highest reported rates occur in countries distant from the equator. Latitude accounts for more than 40% of the geographic variation in rates. Rates have been reported to be higher in Jews.

394. The answer is b. *(Wallace, 14/e, pp 1031–1035.)* Cataract is the main cause of visual loss globally and is the most common eye problem associated with age in the United States, where it can be treated surgically. Risk factors include hypertension, diabetes, exposure to ultraviolet radiation, and corticosteroid therapy. Diabetic retinopathy is less likely to occur in recent onset diabetes, particularly if well controlled. Xerophthalmia refers to blindness due to vitamin A deficiency. Age-related macular degeneration is the leading cause of blindness for persons over the age of 65 in the United States. Prevalence is estimated to be from 6 to 16%. Its pathophysiology is not well understood.

395. The answer is d. *(Wallace, 14/e, p 1073.)* Neurofibromatosis is an autosomal dominant disease, with a 50% probability of transmission to the child. If this child does not have the disease, then she does not have the gene. If she does not have the gene and her partner is asymptomatic, therefore without the gene, then they have 0% probability of transmitting the disease to their child.

396. The answer is b. *(Wallace, 14/e, p 1072.)* Down syndrome, or trisomy 21, is the most common recognizable cause of mental retardation in the Western world. It occurs approximately in 1 out of 1000 births and is strongly correlated with the age of the mother. It is not an inherited disease. Sex chromosome disorders include Turner's syndrome, occurring in girls in 1/5000 births, and Klinefelter's syndrome (an extra X chromosome), occurring in males in 1/500 births. These are generally not associated with significant mental retardation. X-linked recessive disorders include Duchenne's muscular dystrophy and hemophilia. X-linked dominant disorders are rare and include Alport's syndrome. Tay-Sachs disease and cystic fibrosis (1 in 22 white persons carries this gene) are examples of autosomal recessive disorders.

397. The answer is a. *(Wallace, 14/e, pp 1096–1099.)* Although all the measures mentioned are important on an individual basis to reduce caries, fluoridation is the single most cost-effective, safe, and practical public health method to reduce dental caries. No associations have been found with cancer. Fluorosis has been found to be increasing in communities with or without fluoridated water. It is primarily an aesthetic problem. The CDC has estimated that for each dollar spent on water fluoridation, $80 are saved in dental treatment.

398–401. The answers are 398-c, 399-e, 400-b, 401-a. *(Fauci, 14/e [full text], pp 480–486.)* Scurvy due to vitamin C deficiency is characterized by pain and tenderness of the extremities, irritability, and hemorrhagic phenomena, all the result of defective formation of collagen. Niacin deficiency causes pellagra, which results in the four Ds: disturbances of the gastrointestinal tract (diarrhea), of the skin (dermatitis), and of the nervous system (delirium and dementia). Thiamine deficiency leads to beriberi in which either myocardial disease, edema, and cardiac failure or neurological signs predominate. Vitamin A deficiency leads to defects in epithelial cells of skin (hyperkeratosis) and to eye disorders (xerosis and keratomalacia, as well as night blindness). Vitamin D deficiency causes rickets in children and osteomalacia in adults; both conditions are due to the inadequate mineralization of bone.

402–404. The answers are 402-e, 403-a, 404-b. *(Wallace, 14/e, pp 811–814.)* Health belief model: the likelihood of taking a health action is determined by the perceived susceptibility, severity, benefits, and barriers. The social learning theory: behavior change and maintenance are a function of expectations about the outcomes that will result from engaging in a behavior (outcomes expectations) and expectations about one's ability to engage in or execute the behavior (efficacy expectations). The theory of planned behavior (or reasoned action): variables important in determining whether an individual will attempt to perform a behavior include beliefs about the likely consequences of success and failure, the precieved probabilities of success and failure, normative beliefs regarding important referents, and motivation to comply. Stages of change theory is often used in clinical practice (interventions for tobacco cessation).

405–408. The answers are 405-d, 406-a, 407-a, 408-e. *(Wallace, 14/e, p 895. USPS Task Force, 2/e, p xli.)* Primary prevention prevents the occurrence of the condition/disease. Thus, using condoms prevents the acquisition of an STD, and pasteurizing milk prevents brucellosis and other diseases. The treatment of syphilis during pregnancy prevents the infection of the fetus and congenital syphilis, and thus is a primary prevention for the newborn. Treating the mother also prevents the complications of untreated syphilis, such as neurosyphilis, and thus is a measure of tertiary prevention for the mother. Secondary prevention measures are used to detect and treat disease before it becomes clinically manifest. Screening for hypertension in asymptomatic persons is both a secondary measure and a primary measure as it also prevents the occurrence of strokes.

409–412. The answers are 409-e, 410-d, 411-a, 412-c. *(Fauci, 14/e [full text], pp 490–492.)* Fluorine is found in water, seafoods, and plant and animal foods depending upon the concentration of fluorine in the soil and water. It is retained when the intake is 0.6 mg/day and it is excreted in urine and sweat. Supplementation for infants and children in areas without fluoridation of public water supplies is recommended. Copper has many functions. It is a catalyst in hemoglobin formation, essential in production of red blood cells, and required for absorption of iron. The highest concentration is in the liver and central nervous system. It is excreted mainly via the intestinal wall and bile. Good dietary sources of copper are liver, oysters, meats, fish, and whole grains.

Zinc is a constituent of enzymes involved in carbon dioxide exchange and hydrolysis of protein. It is found in liver, bones, and red and white blood cells and is excreted mainly from the intestine. Children have a higher tissue concentration of zinc than adults.

Sodium helps to maintain cellular osmotic pressure, acid-base balance, and muscle and nerve function. It is absorbed easily from the intestine and excreted in the urine and sweat. It is coupled with chloride in many biochemical processes. Table salt, milk, eggs, seasonings, and preservatives are dietary sources of sodium.

Calcium is required for growth of bones and teeth, muscle contraction, nerve irritability, coagulation of blood, cardiac action, and production of milk. It is absorbed from the small intestine with the help of vitamin D. Most is excreted in the feces; the amount retained depends upon the growth rate. Good dietary sources include dairy products, green leafy vegetables, canned salmon, clams, and oysters.

413–415. The answers are 413-b,f,h, 414-c,d,e, 415-c,h. *(Wallace, 14/e, p 824. Fauci, 14/e [full text], pp 563, 568, 605–609.)* Moderate alcohol consumption appears to be a risk factor also for breast cancer. Tobacco use is also associated with cancer of the lip, oral cavity, pharynx, pancreas, larynx, bladder, and kidney.

416–418. The answers are 416-e, 417-a, 418-b. *(USPS Task Force, 2/e, pp lxi–lxix.)* These age groups are based on the USPS Task Force age-specific tables for the periodic health examination (1996).

419–422. The answers are 419-b, 420-f, 421-g, 422-e. *(Fauci, 14/e [full text], pp 647–648, 1448.)* Certain populations are at higher risk of certain diseases and screening programs for genetic diseases should be targeted accordingly. Beta-thalassemias are very common in many parts of southern Europe. In Sardinia, up to 12% of the population have thalassemia traits. Ashkenazic Jews from Poland and Russia are at increased risk of a variety of genetic diseases, including Tay-Sachs disease and Gaucher disease. Persons of African origin are at an increased risk of sickle cell disease (hemoglobin S): up to 7.8% of African Americans have sickle cell traits and 2.3% have hemoglobin C trait. Caucasians from North America are at higher risk of cystic fibrosis (1/300 live births versus 1/17,000 for African Americans and 1/90,000 for Asians in Hawaii). Hemophilia is seen in all ethnic groups. Hemoglobin E is more prevalent in Southeast Asia.

423–424. The answers are 423-a, 424-b. *(Wallace, 14/e, pp 1189–1190.)* The effectiveness of a contraceptive can be evaluated for "perfect use" and "typical use," the latter taking into account compliance issues. Perfect use failure rate of oral contraceptives approaches 0%. However, they must be taken consistently and correctly to achieve this level of effectiveness. Taking this into account provides the "typical" failure rate (failure rate for typical use). Because the IUD is not user-dependent, the typical failure rate and the perfect use failure rate are almost the same and are very low (0.8%). Failure rates of condoms (12%), spermicides (21%), diaphragms (18%), and cervical caps are largely determined by user determinants.

PROVISION OF HEALTH SERVICES

Questions

DIRECTIONS: Each item below contains a question or an incomplete statement followed by suggested responses. Select the **one best** response to each question.

425. Which of the following health measures has the greatest potential for prevention of disease in the United States?

a. Environmental modification
b. Genetic counseling
c. Immunization
d. Modification of personal health behavior
e. Screening tests

426. The largest proportion of the nation's *hospital* bill is covered by

a. Medicare
b. Medicaid
c. Private insurance
d. Other private payers
e. Out-of-pockets payments

Items 427–428

A newly appointed medical director of a federally funded community health center conducts a chart review to examine the immunization rates of the children who are patients at the center. Only 80% of children age 2 have received their basic immunization series.

427. Which of the following is likely to be the most important cause of underimmunization?

a. Parent refusal
b. Provider refusal
c. Lack of insurance coverage
d. Missed opportunities
e. Inadequate number of health supervision visits

428. Which of the following interventions is likely to be most effective in increasing immunization rates?

a. A recall/reminder system
b. A provider education initiative
c. A communitywide education program
d. A one-day immunization event
e. Family incentives

429. A 50-year-old diabetic patient needs to start hemodialysis because of end-stage renal disease. He is entitled to Social Security benefits, but he has no medical insurance. His medical services will be covered by

a. Medicaid
b. The hospital where he receives treatment
c. Medicare
d. Out-of-pocket payments
e. Disability insurance

430. Which of the following programs is responsible for the largest state health department expenditure?

a. HIV/AIDS
b. Maternal and child health
c. Substance abuse
d. Environmental health
e. Chronic diseases

431. Which of the following categories of service accounted for the largest proportion of U.S. health care costs in the 1990s?

a. Hospitals
b. Nursing homes
c. Physicians
d. Dentists
e. Drugs

432. Which of the following determinants is associated with the highest increase in the average length of stay in acute care hospitals?

a. South region of the United States
b. Male gender
c. Age more than 75 years
d. Low socioeconomic status
e. African American race

433. A 75-year-old widowed patient with multiple health problems and limited mobility is in need of nursing home care. Which of the following will be the first source of payment for these services?

a. Medicare
b. Disability insurance
c. Medicaid
d. Patient's financial resources
e. Nursing home

434. Peer Review Organizations (PRO) were initially developed to review care for

a. Medicaid patients
b. Medicare patients
c. All hospitalized patients
d. Health Maintenance Organization (HMO) patients
e. Nursing home patients

435. The National Committee for Quality Assurance (NCQA) was created to accredit which of the following organizations?

a. Health Maintenance Organizations (HMOs)
b. Hospitals
c. Laboratories
d. Nursing homes
e. Pharmacies

436. The resource-based relative value scale (RBRVS) was adopted in 1989 as a payment schedule for Medicare providers to address the imbalance between cognitive services and procedures. Which of the following factors is NOT part of this methodology?

a. Physician time and mental effort
b. Physician skill and judgment
c. Practice expenses
d. Malpractice costs
e. Hospital costs

437. A 65-year-old patient becomes eligible for Medicare benefits. Which of the following services will be covered under this plan?

a. Hearing aids
b. Eyeglasses
c. Clinical laboratory services
d. Dental care
e. Routine physical examinations

438. The majority of uninsured persons in the United States are

a. Unemployed individuals and their families
b. Individuals on public assistance and their families
c. Working individuals and their families
d. Disabled individuals and their families
e. Poor, homeless individuals and their families

439. Which of the following statements best describes Medicare?

a. Medicare is a federal and state cooperative program
b. Medicare includes three parts: A, B, and C
c. Part A of Medicare is financed by premiums from beneficiaries
d. Part B of Medicare is reimbursed using the diagnosis-related groups (DRGs)
e. Anyone over the age of 65 or who is permanently disabled is eligible for coverage under Medicare

440. Total health expenditures in the United States are much higher than in other advanced industrialized nations. In 1993, health spending represented what percentage of the U.S. gross domestic product?

a. 1%
b. 3%
c. 6%
d. 10%
e. 14%

441. The number of Americans without health insurance coverage is estimated to be

a. 1 million
b. 15 million
c. 30 million
d. 45 million
e. 60 million

442. What proportion of total expenditures for health care in the 1990s was covered by governmental programs?

a. 20%
b. 30%
c. 40%
d. 50%
e. 60%

443. Which of the following statements best describes Medicaid?

a. Medicaid is financed only by states
b. Medicaid does not finance long-term care for the elderly
c. Medicaid is required to cover only inpatient hospital services
d. Medicaid provides medical assistance for all poor persons
e. Many states have implemented Medicaid-managed care programs

444. Which of the following methods is the least likely to be effective in controlling costs in managed care organizations?

a. Gatekeeping
b. Utilization review
c. Referral authorization
d. Capitation compensation
e. Fee-for-service compensation

445. Which of the following statements best describes diagnosis-related groups (DRGs)?

a. The DRG is used to provide the reimbursement rates for part B of Medicare
b. The DRG classification system considers the severity of illness
c. The DRG payment system was put into place to stem rising hospital costs
d. Manipulating the system by upgrading the DRG to get the highest possible reimbursement for an admission is called "churning"
e. The DRG is based on the lowest production cost by the most efficient hospital

446. Which of the following statements best describes total quality management (TQM)?

a. It focuses on individuals
b. It seeks to reduce variations in the delivery of services
c. It is provider-focused
d. It relies on expert opinion
e. It seeks to eliminate "bad apples" in order to improve the overall quality of the services

447. Health benefits and costs incurred in the future are often less valued than if they occur today. To take this into consideration, which of the following methods is used in calculations for cost-benefit analysis?

a. Depreciation
b. Amortization
c. Discounting
d. Cost-shifting
e. Utilization

448. An analysis of cost-effectiveness discloses that hemodialysis for a 50-year-old patient costs about $30,000 to $35,000 per quality-adjusted life year (QALY) saved. This indicates that

a. Hemodialysis is not cost-effective
b. Hemodialysis results in a relatively low quality of life
c. Placing a patient with renal failure on dialysis increases his or her life expectancy
d. The annual incremental cost of hemodialysis is more than $40,000
e. Life expectancy of a patient on hemodialysis is less than 20 years

449. Which of the following factors should NOT be considered for implementation of a screening test?

a. Burden of suffering
b. Cost of screening test
c. The physician's familiarity with the disease
d. Potential adverse effects of screening test
e. Efficacy of treatment

450. Which of the following changes occurred in managed care organizations during the 1990s?

a. Growth of staff model Health Maintenance Organizations (HMOs)
b. Decreased use of clinical practice guidelines
c. Declining hospital use
d. Ability to control cost of drugs
e. Increased financial stability

451. According to the Council on Graduate Medical Education (COGME), there will be a shortage of which medical specialty in the coming years?

a. Obstetrics and gynecology
b. Emergency medicine
c. Anesthesiology
d. Ophthalmology
e. Geriatric medicine

452. Which region of the United States has the largest penetration of managed care as a form of health insurance?

a. Northeast
b. Midwest
c. Southeast
d. West
e. Virgin Islands

453. Which of the following statements best describes the trend in group practices in the United States?

a. Group practice offers only cost containment advantages
b. There continues to be a dramatic growth in the number of physicians who are in group practices
c. Multispecialty group practices are the most common type of group practice
d. Most group practices contain more than 15 physicians
e. HMOs do not contract with group practices to provide services

454. *Healthy People 2010*, a document issued by the Department of Health and Human Services, provides a nationwide health promotion and disease prevention agenda. Which of the following are the two goals for *Healthy People 2010*?

a. Increase quality of years and healthy life and eliminate health disparities
b. Increase the proportion of Americans insured and decrease infant mortality rate
c. Decrease the number of preventable hospitalizations and increase research in cancer prevention
d. Decrease poverty and air pollution
e. Increase public health efforts and decrease injuries

455. Because of the aging of the population, provision of long-term care represents one of the challenges of the future. Which of the following statements currently reflects the status of this type of care?

a. There are more male than female patients in nursing homes
b. There is an increasing trend toward larger facilities
c. Home health services are the most costly component of long-term care
d. These services are adequately financed
e. There is an increasing trend toward government ownership

Items 456–458

Match each description below with the proper health care organization.

a. Professional Review Organization (PRO)
b. Health Maintenance Organization (HMO)
c. Independent Practice Association (IPA)
d. Preferred Provider Organization (PPO)
e. Staff model HMO

456. Group of providers who agree to provide services to specific groups of patients on a discounted fee-for-service basis.

457. An organization that directly provides or arranges for all health services required by a defined population of prepaid clients.

458. An organization that contracts with private physicians in the community to provide services to members of prepaid group health plans.

Items 459–461

Match the following programs with the appropriate federal government program.

a. Title V of the Social Security Act
b. Title X of the Public Health Service
c. Title XIX of the Social Security Act
d. Title XVIII of the Social Security Act
e. Title XXI of the Social Security Act

459. Medicaid.

460. Medicare.

461. Maternal and Child Health.

Items 462–465

For each function or program, select the responsible agency.

a. Food and Drug Administration
b. Department of Agriculture
c. Centers for Disease Control and Prevention
d. National Institutes of Health
e. Labor Department
f. Health Resources and Services Administration
g. Office of Health Promotion and Disease Prevention
h. National Center for Health Statistics
i. Occupational Safety and Health Administration (OSHA)

462. Epidemiology and control of injury.

463. Standards for drug manufacturing.

464. Women, Infants, and Children (WIC) nutrition program.

465. Funding for community health centers.

Items 466–468

Match each organization with the correct description.

a. A private voluntary health agency
b. A federal health agency
c. A professional health organization.
d. An international health agency
e. A health foundation

466. American Public Health Association.

467. American Cancer Society.

468. Pan American Health Organization.

PROVISION OF HEALTH SERVICES

Answers

425. The answer is d. *(USPS Task Force, 2/e, pp lxxv–xxx.)* Although environmental modification, genetic counseling, immunization, and screening tests are important elements of preventive health, changing personal health behavior has the largest potential for improving public health in the United States, where the leading causes of death include heart disease, cancer, AIDS, injuries, and chronic obstructive pulmonary disease. Thus, alterations in personal health behaviors—such as smoking, diet, exercise, use of seatbelts, and safe sexual behavior—need to be stressed. Priorities would be different in developing countries where infectious disease and malnutrition are leading causes of death.

426. The answer is c. *(Wallace, 14/e, pp 1116–1118.)* Private insurance pays for 35% of the nation's total hospital bill. Medicare covers 27% and Medicaid, 11%. Out-of-pocket payments account for 5% and other private insurance covers 5.5%, with the remainder provided from a variety of sources.

427–428. The answers are 427-d, 428-a. *(NVAC, JAMA 282:363–370, 1999. CDC, MMWR 48[RR-8]: 1–15, 1999.)* Parental and provider attitudes toward immunization are not barriers for the majority of underimmunized children. Children whose private health insurance does not cover immunizations are entitled to the federal Vaccines for Children (VFC) program at federally qualified health centers. Children on Medicaid or who are uninsured are covered by VFC. Children often fall behind because the parents do not know when the immunizations are due. Making the number of required health supervision visits does not guarantee adequate immunization, and missed opportunities abound because of failure to assess immunization status. Provider practices play a critical role in underimmunization. Providers often overestimate the immunization rates in their practices. They may have no system to identify underimmunized children and have no recall/

reminder system. There is sufficient evidence demonstrating that the implementation of a recall/reminder system, provider-based tracking, and the performance of practice-based immunization assessments with feedback results are effective in increasing immunization rates. These methods are strongly recommended. There is insufficient evidence demonstrating effectiveness to recommend the other methods.

429. The answer is c. *(Wallace, 14/e, pp 965–966.)* The End-Stage Renal Disease (ESRD) Program is funded through Medicare and was enacted in 1971. Eligibility requirements include having ESRD, applying for benefits, and (1) being fully insured for old age and survivor insurance benefits, or (2) entitlement to Social Security benefits, or (3) being a spouse or a dependent of a person who fits the description of 1 or 2. About 93% of all persons with ESRD are eligible. The expenditure for this program far exceeds the initial estimates because many more persons than expected are now receiving the benefits.

430. The answers is b. *(Scutchfield, p 82.)* Based on 1989 data, published in 1991, the largest categories of expense in descending order were maternal and child health, environmental health, substance abuse, HIV/AIDS, and chronic diseases.

431. The answer is a. *(Wallace, 14/e, p 1124.)* Hospital costs accounted for 36.8% of national health expenditures in the United States in 1990 and 35.7% in 1994. Although this represents a decline compared to 1980, when the proportion was 41.5%, this is still almost twice as much as the cost of physician services (19.9%). The proportions of costs devoted to nursing homes, drugs, and dentists were 7.6, 8.3, and 4.4%, respectively.

432. The answer is c. *(Wallace, 14/e, p 1126.)* Older age (≥75 years) is associated with the highest average length of stay (ALOS) in acute care hospitals (8.4 days). Males tend to have longer lengths of stay than females (7.0 versus 5.6 days). There is little difference between African Americans and Caucasians (6.7 versus 6.1 days). Socioeconomic status is inversely related to ALOS. The Northeast region of the United States tends to have longer ALOS (7.6 days) compared to the other regions of the United States (5.8 days for the Midwest, 5.9 days for the South, and 6.3 days for the West).

433. The answer is d. *(Wallace, 14/e, p 1121.)* Medicare does not generally cover nursing home expenses, and so patients must rely on their own resources until they are depleted, at which time they will be covered by Medicaid. Government remains the payer of last resort.

434. The answer is b. *(Wallace, 14/e, p 1118.)* This a federally mandated program to review care provided for patients entitled to Medicare benefits for appropriateness of use.

435. The answer is a. *(Wallace, 14/e, p 1128. Pozgar, 7/e, p 216.)* NCQA is the accreditation body of HMOs. They are also responsible for developing the Health Employers Data and Information Set (HEDIS), a set of quality indicators in the delivery of health care, many points of which assess the performance in the provision of preventive services such as immunization, mammography, and Pap smear screening rates. Hospitals are accredited by JACOH, the Joint Commission on Accreditation of Health Organizations. If a hospital loses its accreditation, it would be grounds for third-party reimbursement agencies, such as Medicare, to refuse payment. Laboratories are generally accredited by the CAP, the College of American Pathologists.

436. The answer is e. *(Wallace, 14/e, p 1125.)* The RBRVS is a system for making doctors' fees more equitable—it does not address hospital costs. It is meant to replace the "usual and customary rate" (UCR) schedule, which strongly rewarded technical procedures at the expense of cognitive services. The practical effect is to lower the reimbursement for procedures such as repair of inguinal hernia and bypass surgery, and to increase reimbursement for an office visit. Family physicians would see an overall increase of 16% while thoracic surgeons would see a decrease of 55%. Proponents hope that the scale will discourage overuse of procedures and encourage physicians to spend more time with their patients.

437. The answer is c. *(Wallace, 14/e, p 1128.)* Medicare does not cover preventive health services (except for mammography), routine medical visits, any services not related to the treatment of an illness or an injury, hearing aids, eyeglasses, dentures, and dental care. Medicare will pay for 100% of the approved amount for medically necessary clinical laboratory services. For other services covered by part B Medicare, such as outpatient hospital treatment, outpatient physician's medical and surgical services, and medical supplies, copayments and deductibles apply. Because of the limited coverage provided by part B and the substantial beneficiary disbursement for some services, more elderly have decided to enroll in managed care plans that cover more services and have lower copayments and deductibles.

438. The answer is c. *(Wallace, 14/e, p 1126.)* Contrary to the belief of many, the majority of the uninsured in the United States are working. They do not have health insurance because they choose not to purchase it or they cannot afford it; many times, it is not offered where they work. Over 85% of all uninsured are working Americans and their families. Many who are insured have limited coverage, often restricted to hospital care.

439. The answer is e. *(Scutchfield, pp 64–65.)* Medicaid is a collaborative federal and state program. Medicare is a federal program with two parts: A and B. Part A covers mostly hospital-related expenses and part B covers physician expenses. Part A is financed by an employee/employer tax, which is paid into a trust fund, while part B is financed partly through beneficiary premiums and partly from the U.S. general fund budget. Part A is reimbursed using DRGs, and part B is moving from "usual, customary, and prevailing reimbursement" to the resource-based relative value scale (RBRVS). Medicare covers persons over the age of 65 or those who are permanently disabled.

440. The answer is e. *(Wallace, 14/e, p 1124.)* The United States spends much more money on health care than any other industrialized country in the world. In 1993, total health expenditure as a percent of the gross national product was 13.6% in the United States, 10.2% in Canada, 9.9% in Switzerland, and 7.1% in the United Kingdom. This proportion has been gradually rising in the United States, from 5.1% in 1960. Reasons for this increase include the aging of the population, the technological advances, and the increase in insurance coverage.

441. The answer is d. *(USDHHS, Healthy People 2010, 1999.)* More than 44 million Americans have no health insurance at all. Tens of millions more are underinsured, often with hefty deductibles and copayments or coverage only for inpatient acute services. Even those who have insurance face losing it if they change their employment.

442. The answer is c. *(Wallace, 14/e, p 1124.)* The largest payer of medical expenses is the government (40%), followed by private insurance (33%). Out-of-pocket expenditures accounted for 20% and all other sources constituted 5%.

443. The answer is e. *(Wallace, 14/e, p 1128.)* Medicaid is financed by both the federal and state governments. In order to receive federal funds, states are required to provide certain basic benefits such as inpatient and outpatient hospital services, family planning services and supplies, and to cover certain groups such as recipients of supplemental security income and Aid to Families with Dependent Children (AFDC). However, states do not cover *all* poor persons, and coverage will vary from state to state. Seventy-five percent of all Medicaid expenditures for the elderly went to pay for nursing home services. Medicaid will cover these services once a person has spent down to an eligibility level.

444. The answer is e. *(Gabel, Health Affairs 16:134–144, 1997.)* Measures to control costs in HMOs include gatekeeping, which means that a person is assigned to a primary care provider who coordinates all the care for that person, as well as authorization for referrals and emergency room use. It promotes continuity of care and decreases excessive unnecessary care. However, some plans have abandoned specialist visit referral authorization because analysis showed that they approved over 90% of referrals while incurring large administrative costs (bottom line = no cost savings). Utilization review is used for both cost containment and quality assurance. Authorization by the plan is required for hospitalization and referrals to specialists, and the length of stay in the hospital is monitored. The use of fee-for-service as a method of compensation for physicians actually may encourage more procedures and more services and does not contain costs, let alone decrease them. HMOs are turning to capitation to reduce overutilization. By this method of payment, the physician receives a set amount of money to care for each patient who is assigned to him or her. Effective monitoring and quality assurance mechanisms must be in place to guard against underutilization with this form of payment. However, only capitation has proved to stabilize, if not reduce, health care costs.

445. The answer is c. *(Wallace, 14/e, p 1128.)* The DRG is used to calculate the reimbursement rate for part A of Medicare. This system was created to stem the rising costs of hospital care. A fixed amount of money is given to the hospital for the diagnosis for which the patient was hospitalized. This is calculated based on the average costs of a large number of hospitals to care for someone with a particular diagnosis. It is not based on the costs associated with the most efficient care, and it does not take into account severity of illness. For any hospital, the actual cost may be higher or lower than the DRG payment. Upgrading the DRG to obtain a higher reimbursement is called "DRG creep"; *churning* is readmitting the patient several times for related procedures or diagnoses, which results in additional DRG payments.

446. The answer is b. *(Scutchfield, pp 133–134.)* The principle of TQM was introduced by W. E. Deming and was initially applied to industrial management. The basis is to be customer-focused, to use data to better understand variations, and to work on improving the process of delivery. The belief is that most errors and less-than-optimal outcomes occur because of systemic problems rather than because individuals are poorly motivated or incompetent. A team approach is used to work on improving a process. The "plan-do-check-act" strategy is then applied. Individuals are helped to improve their performance (as opposed to being singled out as in the elimination of the "bad apple"). The analogy often used is that TQM tries to move to a higher level the mean of a normal distribution rather than to cut out the tail values (which quality assurance does). This approach is now increasingly used in medical management.

447. The answer is c. *(Fauci, 14/e [companion volume], pp 50–51.)* *Discounting* is the term used to describe the reduced value of money and benefits first realized in the future. It is dependent on monetary inflation (one dollar is worth more today than in five years), as well as on the extent to which society wishes to invest today's dollars for future health (health today is more valued than health in 20 years). Depreciation and amortization refer to the process by which capital investments are written off over a period of years. Cost-shifting occurs when the costs of care for some people, usually poor and uninsured, are shifted to others who are able to pay the bills.

448. The answer is c. *(Fauci, 14/e, pp 50–51.)* Hemodialysis must increase life expectancy, otherwise it would result in a situation in which there is cost per year of life lost. Quality-adjusted life years (QALYs) are an attempt to compare the value of life in the presence of a chronic medical problem such as the need for hemodialysis with perfect health, which is assigned a value of 1.0; the quality adjustment for patients on hemodialysis would differ among patients, but would be less than 1.0—perhaps, say, 0.9. In its most simple formulation, cost per QALY saved is simply cost divided by the quality adjustment. Thus, cost is cost-effectiveness multiplied by the quality adjustment, and the cost of hemodialysis, since the quality adjustment is less than 1.0, must be less than $30,000 to $35,000 per year. There is no way to determine life expectancy or quality of life in this situation, nor can one ever say whether a technology is cost-effective unless one asks against what its cost-effectiveness is to be compared.

449. The answer is c. *(USPS Task Force, 2/e, pp xxvii–xxxiii.)* A variety of factors need to be considered before instituting any preventive health measure, including a screening test. The burden of suffering includes both the severity and the prevalence of the disease. Other things being equal, rare diseases are less important than more common diseases, and illnesses of minor clinical significance are less important than illnesses with high morbidity and mortality. Recall also that the positive predictive value of a screening test increases as prevalence of the disease increases. Another requirement for the rational institution of a screening program is the availability both technically and socioeconomically of effective treatment. If no effective intervention is available for a disease, screening will only serve to produce a lead-time bias: an apparent prolongation of life by detecting a disease at an earlier stage without a true impact on survival. Additional criteria for screening tests include cost, efficacy, and potential adverse effects. The ideal screening test is inexpensive and reliable and has high sensitivity and specificity. Low specificity and prevalence lead to many patients with false-positive results, who must then undergo further evaluation and therapy with the attendant risk of iatrogenic morbidity. The targeting of screening tests to populations specifically at risk rather than to the population as a whole will limit costs, reduce the number of false-positives, and hence decrease the adverse effects of screening.

450. The answer is d. *(Gabel, Health Affairs 16:134–144, 1997.)* There are less staff model HMOs in 1999, and there is a growing trend toward independent practice associations (IPAs) and network model HMOs. More physicians are paid through capitation (risk sharing), and there is also increased patient cost sharing. Hospital use has declined, but the use of practice guidelines has increased. There are more HMOs on the verge of financial collapse than ever, due to underpricing, expansion, mergers, inability to control medical costs, particularly drugs, and reduced ability to shift costs to other payers.

451. The answer is e. *(Wallace, 14/e, p 1122.)* According to COGME, there will be a shortage in primary care, geriatric, and preventive medicine. Managed care has emphasized the need for primary care physicians, and there is concern about specialty distribution (excess of specialists).

452. The answer is d. *(Wallace, 14/e, p 1127.)* In 1995, 29% of the population in the West are enrolled in HMOs, compared to 20.9% in the Northeast, 14.4% in the Midwest, and 11.2% in the South. These percentages have been growing in all areas of the United States since 1990.

453. The answer is b. *(Wallace, 14/e, p 1119.)* The American Medical Association conducts surveys about the structure of physician practices in the United States. For a variety of reasons (sharing costs, flexible hours, coverage, interaction, one stop for patients, etc.), there is an increasing trend toward group practices. Most still consist of 10 physicians or less. Multispecialty groups are on the rise.

454. The answer is a. *(USDHHS, Healthy People 2010, 1999.)* The overarching goals of *Healthy People 2010* are to increase the quality and years of healthy life and decrease health disparities. Progress toward achieving these goals will be monitored through 467 objectives in 28 focus areas. Leading health indicators reflect the major public health concerns of the United States. They are the following: physical activity, obesity, tobacco use, substance abuse, responsible sexual behavior, mental health, injury and violence, environmental quality, immunization, and access to health care.

455. The answer is b. *(Wallace, 14/e, pp 1121.)* Residents of nursing homes are predominantly females (since females have a longer life expectancy than males) over the age of 75 who have multiple health problems. Medicaid, not Medicare, covers nursing home costs. Medicare will pay for a limited stay in a skilled nursing facility. Nursing homes usually are paid for "out-of-pocket" until the patient is indigent, and then Medicaid will pay. Nursing home care, not home health services, is the most expensive component of long-term care. While in the past, nursing homes have tended to be small, proprietary operations, there is a move toward larger, multihome systems, either nonprofit or proprietary. Increased financial support would greatly increase access and meeting the needs of the elderly.

456–458. The answers are 456-d, 457-b, 458-c. *(Wallace, 14/e, pp 1126–1128.)* Preferred Provider Organizations (PPOs) are groups of providers that make special arrangements with insurers to provide services to their customers on a discounted basis, that is, to accept lower levels of reimbursement than their usual rates. An example is the Blue Cross Prudent Buyer Plan, in which patients who are willing to obtain care from preferred providers can save on coinsurance and deductibles.

Health Maintenance Organizations (HMOs) provide comprehensive health care services on a prepaid basis. First developed around the turn of the twentieth century, they were bitterly opposed by organized medicine. In the early 1970s, legislation encouraging their development was passed, which led to the establishment of 166 HMOs by 1975 and to 323 HMOs covering 15 million members by 1985.

Independent Practice Associations (IPAs) are a more recent development. Whereas HMOs have traditionally served their patients by employing full-time physicians in their own clinics and medical centers, IPAs allow private physicians to contract with HMOs to provide services to enrolled patients.

Professional Review Organizations (PROs) are federally mandated programs to review care provided for patients entitled to Medicare benefits for appropriateness of use (see question 434).

Staff model HMOs employ salaried physicians, but these types of HMOs are decreasing in favor of other arrangements discussed previously (IPA, PPO) or mixed-model HMOs.

459–461. The answers are 459-c, 460-d, 461-a. *(Scutchfield, pp 64, 322, 332.)* Passages of titles XVIII and XIX of the Social Securiy Act occurred under President Johnson in 1965, making health care available for many Americans who had been without insurance. Title V of the Social Security Act authorizes the Maternal and Child Health block grant to the states and territories: 30% of their federal allotment must go to provide preventive and primary care health services to children. Title XXI (Children's Health Insurance Program) is used to provide funds to states to enable them to initiate and expand the provision of health coverage for children. Title X is for allocation of funds to provide family planning services.

462–465. The answers are 462-c, 463-a, 464-b, 465-f. (*Scutchfield, pp 59–64.*) The Centers for Disease Control and Prevention (CDC) is responsible for providing disease surveillance; tracing epidemiology and controling infectious diseases, injury, and chronic diseases; promoting disease-control programs; and providing expert laboratory assistance to state and local health departments.

The Food and Drug Administration (FDA) was established in 1906 to enforce the laws that regulated interstate transport and quality of drugs and food. The FDA, which received its current name in 1931, assures that safe and effective prescription drugs are sold to the public. To do this, the FDA tests products, sets standards for production and quality control, and judges claims of safety and efficacy.

The Women, Infants, and Children (WIC) food assistance program is the largest federally funded state health program. It is administered by the U.S. Department of Agriculture and provides supplemental food for pregnant and nursing women, infants, and children.

OSHA is under the Department of Labor and is responsible for workplace safety: it conducts inspections and develops safety standards based on research findings from the National Institute of Occupational Safety and Health (NIOSH). The National Institutes of Health is the largest Public Health Service agency in budgetary terms, with a primary mission of health-related research.

The Office of Health Promotion and Disease Prevention was responsible for developing the *Healthy People 2010* objectives. Tracking activities for meeting the objectives can be achieved by using the data from the National Center for Health Statistics.

The Health Resources and Services Administration (HRSA) funds health profession education (such as support for residents in preventive medicine programs) and community health centers. It houses the National Health Service Corps and other programs aimed at providing health services for underserved areas.

466–468. The answers are 466-c, 467-a, 468-d. (*Scutchfield, pp 101, 235.*) Professional health organizations are groups formed by persons who have met prescribed standards of training and certification and whose purposes are to promote the interests of the profession and to serve the public. An example is the American Public Health Association, founded in 1872, which establishes standards and guidelines related to public health; implements public health education through its journal, other publications, and meetings; and provides expert testimony to legislative groups.

The American Cancer Society, founded in 1913, is an example of a nonprofit, voluntary health agency, which was organized to disseminate knowledge about cancer and is supported by voluntary donations.

The Pan American Health Organization, established in 1901, is an international health agency representing the nations of the Americas. Its major concern has been control of communicable diseases. It has been integrated into the World Health Organization and serves as the regional office for the Americas.

LEGAL AND ETHICAL ISSUES

Questions

DIRECTIONS: Each item below contains a question or incomplete statement followed by suggested responses. Select the **one best** response to each question.

469. *Police power* is defined as the legal authority to protect the health of the public. This power resides in

a. Federal government
b. State government
c. County government
d. Health care providers
e. Individuals

470. A 55-year-old patient suffering from terminal lung cancer is admitted to the hospital for end of life care. Before his admission, he completed a written statement determining his wishes for circumstances of termination of life-sustaining care. This statement represents

a. Advanced directives
b. Power of attorney
c. Do not resuscitate (DNR) order
d. Duty to care
e. Euthanasia

471. One of your patients returns to your office for the results of his HIV test. You inform him that his test is positive for antibodies to HIV. He is married and sexually active with his wife. In the course of subsequent counseling, you tell him it is important that his wife be advised of the exposure. He refuses to tell his wife or have anyone else inform her of the exposure. At this time, what is the most appropriate management of the situation?

a. Tell the patient you refuse to continue seeing him unless his wife is informed
b. Send an anonymous letter to his wife informing her of the exposure
c. Try to convince him of the importance of informing his wife and offer assistance
d. Contact public health authorities so they can inform his wife
e. Call his wife and set up an appointment at your office to inform her of the exposure

472. A 15-year-old girl presents to your office because she has been having vaginal discharge. In the course of the history, she informs you that she is sexually active with her boyfriend who is also 15 years of age. The examination reveals mucopurulent cervicitis, but no lower abdominal, cervical motion or adnexal tenderness. The most appropriate intervention is to

a. Notify the department of social services
b. Obtain parental consent for treatment
c. Provide counseling, testing, and treatment for STDs
d. Refer her to a family planning clinic
e. Notify the department of public health

473. The carelessness or dereliction of duty by a professional person is called

a. Criminal negligence
b. Malfeasance
c. Misfeasance
d. Malpractice
e. Incompetence

474. Which of the following elements is NOT required to be present in order for a patient to recover damages due to negligence?

a. Duty to care
b. Breach of duty
c. Injury
d. Nonfeasance
e. Proximate cause

475. Which of the following patients is incompetent and should receive medical care against his or her expressed wishes?

a. A 32-year-old Jehovah's Witness who had refused transfusions for a ruptured ectopic pregnancy and is now unresponsive postoperatively with a hematocrit of 8%
b. An anxious, frightened 48-year-old patient who refuses surgery for gastric cancer because "it's too scary"
c. A 55-year-old executive with chest pain and ECG changes who refuses hospitalization because of "an important business deal"
d. An active 83-year-old diabetic who refuses treatment for a gangrenous foot ulcer because "I'm going to die anyway"
e. A 25-year-old schizophrenic patient refusing hospitalization because the voices are telling him to continue preaching

476. To obtain informed consent, which of the following is NOT required?

a. Disclosure of the nature and purpose of the proposed therapy
b. Disclosure of the risks and benefits of the proposed therapy
c. Alternatives to the proposed therapy
d. Consequences if the proposed therapy is not given
e. Signature of the patient on the written consent form

477. Which of the following is the major difference between a claims-made policy and an occurrence policy for professional liability insurance?

a. Maximum obligation
b. Requirement for notification of event/claim
c. Type of medical specialty covered
d. Coverage of events prior to the institution of the policy
e. Type of legal defense

478. A physician is invited as a guest speaker to present on the diagnosis and management of sexually transmitted diseases. She receives support from a company that manufactures a drug used for the treatment of chlamydial infections. Which of the following statements reflects the ethical obligations of the presenter toward the conference participants?

a. She should decline the invitation to speak
b. She should disclose only corporate research grants
c. She should disclose only corporate research grants and stock holdings
d. She should not disclose any relationship as there are no standards of ethics in such cases
e. She should disclose research grants, stock holdings, consultant status, and speaker's bureau activities of any company related to products discussed

479. When debating whether providing or withholding medical treatment is ethical, the LEAST important consideration of those listed below is

a. Indications for medical intervention
b. Expected quality of life
c. Patient's preferences
d. Physician's preferences
e. Economic factors

480. A physician calls the state health department because she believes a child she recently vaccinated is experiencing an adverse reaction. She is unsure of the lot number or the batch as she received the vaccine from two different pharmaceutical companies. Which of the following chart documentations of vaccination is required?

a. Type of vaccine and date of administration
b. Type of vaccine, manufacturer, and date of administration
c. Type of vaccine, lot number, manufacturer, and date of administration
d. Type of vaccine, lot number, manufacturer, date of administration, and physician name
e. There are no mandates for chart documentation

481. In the health care setting, who is required to report instances of child sexual abuse?

a. Physicians
b. Social service workers
c. Dentists
d. Psychologists
e. All of these providers

482. Which of the following statements best reflects "Good Samaritan" laws?

a. They have been enacted only by a few states
b. They are designed to encourage health professionals to provide assistance in emergency situations
c. They free providers from liability for gross or criminal negligence
d. They generally require that assistance be rendered with payment or expectation of payment for services
e. They apply only to professionals

483. Which of the following is NOT a medical ethics basic principle?

a. Consent
b. Nonmaleficence
c. Beneficence
d. Justice
e. Respect for autonomy

484. The medical director of a group practice sends an e-mail to his colleagues asking them to refer patients for testing at Lab Incognito Inc. He does not tell them that this laboratory is billing third-party payers and giving him a 10% incentive fee for each bill collected. Which of the following is correct?

a. This practice is acceptable
b. There is no conflict of interest
c. Only Medicare prohibits this type of agreement
d. This type of agreement constitutes a criminal act
e. Disclosure to his colleagues is necessary to continue this practice

485. A physician receives a letter from a patient's attorney claiming alleged injury. She immediately reviews the medical chart of the patient and adds extra data to clarify the situation. Which of the following statements is true?

a. This action is likely to be viewed favorably
b. This action is likely to be used against her
c. This action is never contested in court if comments are dated
d. This action is always recommended by attorneys
e. This action can only include statements to the effect that the patient understood treatment options

486. As organ transplantation has become more common, guidelines have been developed to govern organ donation. The Uniform Anatomical Gift Act does NOT cover which of the following?

a. Allow partial donation
b. Free health care personnel from civil and criminal liability when acting in good faith
c. Limit which physicians may certify time of death
d. Provide for revocation of a donation
e. Require express, documented consent by the donor

487. A surgeon performs surgery on his wife and friends, and prescibes medication to his family members. Which of the statements about this practice is most appropriate?

a. It is illegal in many states
b. Most third-party payers will reimburse for these procedures
c. Professional objectivity may be compromised
d. These procedures will not be covered by the liability insurance
e. Family members cannot sue the surgeon if adverse outcomes occur

488. Which of the following statements is true concerning physicians with substance abuse problems?

a. Physicians are not under any obligation to advise the state medical board
b. Physicians can practice when under the influence of drugs or alcohol
c. Physicians with substance abuse problems always lose their licenses to practice medicine
d. Substance abuse problems such as narcotic abuse are rare in the medical profession
e. Physicians can maintain their licenses if they never practice under the influence and they enter a rehabilitation program

Items 489–492

Match each of the following legal cases with the relevant subject matter.

a. Abortion
b. Duty to warn
c. Informed consent
d. Malpractice liability
e. Termination of life support

489. *Darling* v. *Charleston Community Memorial Hospital.* (**SELECT 1 SUBJECT**)

490. In re *Quinlan.* (**SELECT 1 SUBJECT**)

491. *Tarasoff* v. *Regents of the University of California.* (**SELECT 1 SUBJECT**)

492. *Roe v. Wade.* (SELECT 1 SUBJECT)

Items 493–495

Match the following situations with the appropriate legal claim.

a. Abandonment
b. Assault
c. Battery
d. False imprisonment
e. Misdiagnosis

493. Informed consent is not obtained for a surgical procedure. (SELECT 1 CLAIM)

494. A physician does not follow up after the acute stage of an illness. (SELECT 1 CLAIM)

495. Restraints are used on a competent, nonviolent patient. (SELECT 1 CLAIM)

Items 496–498

Match the following actions to the underlying ethical principle.

a. Autonomy
b. Beneficence
c. Euthanasia
d. Supererogation
e. Utilitarianism

496. A state legislature decides to allocate funds to prenatal care instead of intensive care nurseries. (SELECT 1 PRINCIPLE)

497. A person with AIDS refuses intubation for *Pneumocystis carinii* pneumonia and dies. (SELECT 1 PRINCIPLE)

498. A 27-year-old woman donates a kidney to her 17-year-old brother, who has end-stage renal disease. (SELECT 1 PRINCIPLE)

Items 499–500

Match the following statements with the appropriate legal term.

a. Tort
b. Breach of contract
c. Slander
d. Libel
e. Antitrust

499. Civil wrong against a person or property for which a court provides an action for damages.

500. Written words of defamation.

LEGAL AND ETHICAL ISSUES

Answers

469. The answer is b. *(Potterat, STD 26:345–349, 1999; Richards, STD 26:350–357, 1999.)* Police power resides at the state level. These powers are broad and include any action that seems reasonable to protect the health of the public and prevent epidemics. States have the legal authority to require reporting of disease and to identify infectious disease through screening. Although it is rarely used, states have the power to involuntarily confine an individual to treat an infectious disease if that person refuses treatment and is a threat to the public health. However, this role continues to be controversial in balancing the health of the public and individual rights.

470. The answer is a. *(Fauci, 14/e [full text], pp 6–8. Pozgar, 7/e, pp 493–495, 507–511.)* Advanced directives are statements by competent persons to direct care before they lose decision-making capabilities: they may state which interventions they choose or refuse or they may designate someone who can make those decisions for them. A living will directs caregivers to forego or continue life-sustaining care. Power of attorney allows patients to designate a proxy to make health care decisions for them when they lose that capacity. A DNR is a chart notification to forego resuscitation efforts which must take into account patient autonomy, advanced directives, and underlying medical conditions. Physicians have a duty to care for dying patients with compassion, to relieve suffering, and attend to their psychological distress. Euthanasia refers to the practice of painlessly ending life for persons suffering from incurable conditions. It is defined as active (comission of an act to end life) or passive (withholding life-saving treatment). There is considerable controversy around this issue as well as major ethical and legal issues, but it has not been legalized.

471. The answer is c. *(Pozgar, 7/e, pp 476–477.)* The major issues are confidentiality and duty to warn a third party. When a person initially learns that he or she is HIV-positive, the information in itself is often overwhelming. The patient may not feel capable or willing to inform exposed partners. The best approach is to try to convince the patient of the necessity of this, perhaps at a later visit. Some states have enacted laws to allow the physician to inform third parties of HIV exposure, but *only after efforts by the physician have failed to convince the person to disclose.* These laws protect the physician against legal liability for breach of confidentiality, but they do not obligate the physician to disclose to third parties. Some *few* state laws allows only state disease intervention specialists (DIS) to inform third parties of HIV exposure after the physician has contacted them. *Many states do not have any of these laws,* and the only option is to try to convince an infected patient to disclose. As a rule, for all other STDs, partner notification is *confidential and voluntary,* and the DIS cannot inform third parties without the consent of the infected person, even if requested by the physician. They can assist consenting infected persons in informing contacts either by doing it for them (contacts are *never* informed of the source) or coaching them to do it themselves.

472. The answer is c. *(Pozgar, 7/e, p 406.)* Most states have laws that allow physicians to provide medical services to minors for sexually transmitted diseases without parental consent. Referring to a family planning clinic (where teens can always be seen without parental consent) can be an option, but there is a probability that she will delay (or forego) the visit, resulting in a complicated infection, such as PID. Notifying the department of public health is not necessary, but they could assist you in partner notification, if the patient consents. At the very least, she must be informed that it is crucial that her partner be evaluated and treated. Consensual sexual activity between minors does not need to be reported to social services as cases of statutory rape. Sexual activity with an adult should raise concern about abusive relationships.

473. The answer is d. *(Pozgar, 7/e, pp 38–39.)* Legally, negligence is defined in terms of the expected behavior of a "reasonably prudent person" in a certain situation. Criminal negligence is the reckless disregard for the well-being of another and would usually constitute gross negligence as opposed to ordinary negligence. Malpractice is the negligence of a professional person such as a physician, nurse, or lawyer. Malfeasance is the performance of an unlawful act. Misfeasance is the improper performance of a lawful act that results in injury to another.

474. The answer is d. *(Pozgar, 7/e, p 39.)* Duty to use due care is the legal obligation of one party to protect another party by conforming to a specific standard of care. This duty arises from the doctor-patient, nurse-patient, or hospital-patient relationship and can be created by a telephone call or by displaying an emergency room sign. A physician passing an accident victim on the highway has a moral obligation to stop and render assistance, but there is no legal obligation because the doctor-patient relationship is not established.

Breach of duty is the failure to fulfill this duty according to the prevailing standard of care. Standard of care is based on the behavior of a hypothetical "reasonably prudent person" with similar training and knowledge. This standard may be a national or an "industry" standard as opposed to a community standard. Expert witness testimony is often used in attempts to define this standard.

Unless injuries actually occur, damages cannot be awarded. Malpractice may have been committed, but if there were no untoward results, damages due to negligence cannot be recovered. The legal term *injuries* includes mental anguish and violation of rights and privileges in addition to physical harm.

Finally, causation must be established. This must be a reasonable and close relationship, but it need not be direct. For example, an accident victim who has never encountered the physician may receive damages for physician negligence when injured by a patient who is driving under the influence of a drug prescribed by the physician if the patient received no warnings concerning the drug's intoxicating nature.

Nonfeasance is a negligent act of omission, failing to perform an act that a reasonably prudent person would be expected to perform under the same circumstances. This would satisfy the criteria for breach of duty, but in itself is not necessary for the awarding of damages.

475. The answer is e. *(Pozgar, 7/e, pp 402–407.)* Requirements for competency to refuse or consent to medical treatment include attainment of legal age, the ability to comprehend and communicate information, and the ability to reason and deliberate about one's choices. The legal pronouncement may well require a judicial hearing, which may not be available in clinical emergencies. Patients portrayed in *a* through *d* are presumed competent given the available information. Adherence to religious or unusual beliefs does not make one incompetent. Thus, the wishes of the Jehovah's Witness not to be transfused must be respected since they were expressed at a time when she was competent. Change in medical condition does not alter the power of the original statement. Similarly, affective states such as anxiety or nonpathologic depression do not make a patient incompetent when he or she refuses recommended medical treatment. One is ethically obligated to work with the patient in this situation and to try to explain options in a comforting manner, but patient autonomy still prevails. The elderly diabetic with a foot ulcer and the executive with chest pain are also competent to refuse medical treatment, for each is capable of understanding information and making a deliberate decision. Decision-making capacity is impaired by psychotic episodes in mentally impaired patients.

476. The answer is e. (*Fauci, 14/e [full text], pp 4–6.*) To make an informed decision regarding treatment, patients need to be informed not only of the risks of the treatment, but also of its expected efficacy and the expected efficacy and risks of alternative treatments. Consent should be obtained before sedation, not only because the discussion should take place while the patient is lucid, but also because sedation itself may be associated with risks. Consent may be obtained verbally, but it is best to note in the chart that the conversation took place. As a general rule, the need to inform patients of adverse effects of treatment is more dependent on the severity of the adverse effect than on its frequency. Written consent is not always required, although it is done for most major interventions. It provides proof that some degree of dialogue occurred between a health care provider and a patient, but it is not an absolute protection against liability or proof that the information was understood.

477. The answer is d. (*Pozgar, 7/e, pp 541–542.*) Professional liability insurance policies' malpractice coverage includes provisions for an insurance agreement, defense and settlement, the policy period, the amount payable, and the conditions of the policy. The policy period varies according to the type of insurance policy. An *occurrence* policy covers all incidents that take place during the year the policy is in effect, regardless of when they are reported or when legal action is initiated (given that the statute of limitations has not expired). Advantages of this form of insurance include continued coverage beyond the time period during which premiums are paid. For example, under this type of policy a retired physician would still be covered for events that occurred during active practice. In contrast, the *claims-made* policy covers only those claims made or reported during the policy year. Insurance companies worry about assuming liability for events that occurred prior to the initiation of the policy, and physicians must worry about ongoing coverage after the policy expires.

Malpractice policies cover professional liability only and contain limitations on the amount of damages covered. Policies usually contain a maximum for any individual claim as well as a limit to aggregate claims. Amounts awarded in excess of the insurance limit must be provided for by the individual professional. The insurance company agrees to provide a defense for the insured against lawsuits in which the attorney's obligations are to the insured professional directly, not to the insurance company. However, insurance companies often retain the power to effect a settlement, in which cases the attorney has responsibilities to the insurance company as well.

All insurance policies contain important provisions with which the physician must comply to keep the policy in effect, regardless of the policy period. These include requirements for prompt notification of occurrence and claim and a duty to assist the insurance company to reach a settlement. Other provisions govern relationships with other insurance companies, shared liability, and the terms of change or cancellation of the policy.

478. The answer is e. *(AMA, ACCME, 1999.)* The Accreditation Council for Continuing Medical Education (ACCME) of the American Medical Association has set strict standards for speaker disclosure of corporate affiliation as well as for how corporate contributions can be used to support conferences. If a speaker has some form of corporate relationship, it must be disclosed to the participants, even if it is not meant to imply that bias is present.

479. The answer is d. *(English, pp 98–10. Fauci, 14/e [full text], p 7.)* The overriding consideration in questions of clinical ethics is the patient's preference, which reflects the principle of autonomy. In most cases, physicians are morally obligated to respect the patient's wishes, and strong efforts to identify the patient's preferences must be made. Another important general category for consideration is the indication for medical intervention. Physicians need to make objective, educated judgments about the risks and benefits of diagnostic and therapeutic efforts. Measures that clearly are not medically indicated need not be pursued, even in the face of a patient's preference. Examples here include do not resuscitate (DNR) orders and termination of ineffective therapy in terminally ill patients. Considerations of quality of life include elements of the patient's preference, disease progression, and efficacy of treatment. If the patient's preferences are known, they are overriding. More often, considerations of quality of life become important in situations in which the patient is incompetent to make decisions and no preference has been voiced previously. Economic considerations are becoming more and more important as health care resources become more scarce and decisions are made about the rationing and allocation of health care dollars. These considerations are very important in expensive, high-technology measures such as organ transplant and intensive care.

The physician's preferences are relatively unimportant in ethical decisions. Objective medical judgment is a critical input as described previously, but subjective preference of the physician yields consistently to the patient's preference. However, physicians need not be compelled to act in ways contrary to their own ethical beliefs. For example, an obstetrician cannot be forced to perform abortions or an oncologist forced to provide ongoing chemotherapy for a patient with a terminal, end-stage illness. The physician does, however, have an obligation to assist a patient in finding a new provider who is able to work with the patient.

480. The answer is d. *(Fauci, 14/e [full text], p 762.)* The National Childhood Vaccine Injury Act (NCVIA) of 1986, amended in 1995, requires that all mandated childhood vaccinations be recorded by the health care providers in the permanent medical record.

481. The answer is e. *(Pozgar, 7/e, pp 419–420.)* Persons in the health care setting who are required to report suspected cases of child abuse include physicians, registered nurses, chiropractors, social service workers, psychologists, dentists, osteopaths, optometrists, podiatrists, mental health professionals, and volunteers in residential facilities. Many statutes also specifically include hospital administrators. Most states provide for a variety of civil and criminal penalties for failure to report child abuse incidents.

482. The answer is b. *(Pozgar, 7/e, p 39.)* Good Samaritan laws free health professionals from ordinary negligence in emergency situations where no preexisting duty to use due care exists. They do not apply to acute situations in the emergency room, but rather are designed to encourage health professionals to volunteer their assistance in emergency situations by eliminating liability concerns. No expectation of financial compensation can exist, for this implies a professional/contractual relationship. Good Samaritan laws have been enacted by almost all states, but statutes vary; they may apply for lay persons as well. While the law frees providers from liability for ordinary negligence, it does not free persons from liability for gross or criminal negligence, or from "willful or wanton" misconduct.

483. The answer is a. *(Wallace, 14/e, p 35.)* Medical ethics is founded on four principles. Respect for autonomy is the concern for individual rights. Each person has the right to make decisions about his or her own care. Part of this decision making requires the provision of sufficient information for informed consent. *Primum non nocere,* first do no harm, is also a basic principle of medical ethics (nonmaleficence). Beneficence is the principle of doing good, and justice refers to equity in delivering medical services.

484. The answer is d. *(Pozgar, 7/e, p 100.)* This type of "kickback" practice is specifically prohibited by law under any circumstances and constitutes a criminal act punishable under federal and state laws by fines and/or imprisonment. Medicare has a specific law with a fine of not more than $25,000 or imprisonment of not more than five years or both.

485. The answer is b. *(Pozgar, 7/e, pp 93, 387–388.)* Adding data to the chart, backdated or not, may be construed as falsification of data, which is grounds for criminal prosecution and civil liability. It certainly violates standard of care. The best approach is to never alter a chart under any circumstances.

486. The answer is e. *(Pozgar, 7/e, pp 529–531.)* The Uniform Anatomical Gift Act permits persons 18 years of age or older to donate their body or parts of their body to medical education, science, or transplantation. The person must be of sound mind and the donation should be made by will or other written instrument. However, if the deceased has made no statements objecting to donation, a donation may still be made if relatives or guardians consent. This consent should be recorded. A donation may be revoked by written or oral means, with specific criteria for witnesses. Persons acting in good faith are not liable for criminal or civil negligence when participating in organ donation unless there has been notice of revocation of donation. This is designed to remove obstacles for participation in organ transplantation procedures and is similar to Good Samaritan laws. To eliminate conflict of interest and the overzealous harvesting of organs, time of death of the donor cannot be certified by any physician involved in the transplant procedure.

487. The answer is c. *(AMA, Committee on Ethical and Judicial Affairs, 2000.)* Although there are no specific laws prohibiting this practice, physicians should not treat themselves or members of their immediate family, unless it is an emergency or an isolated setting where no other qualified physician is available. There are situations in which routine short-term care may be appropriate, but physicians should not play the role of the regular primary care provider. Except in emergencies, it is not appropriate for physicians to write prescriptions for controlled substances for themselves or their family members.

488. The answer is e. *(Fauci, 14/e, pp 250–2510; AMA, Committee on Ethical and Judicial Affairs, 2000.)* Reporting is mandated by state medical boards. Physicians should not practice under the influence. Physicians, nurses, and pharmacists are the second group, after patients with chronic pain syndromes, at highest risk of opioid dependence because of easy access. Because of growing awareness of these problems, impaired physician programs have been established in hospitals and state medical societies to help physicians abstain before licensure revocation occurs.

489–492. The answers are 489-d, 490-e, 491-b, 492-a. *(Pozgar, 7/e, pp 208–209, 284–285, 433–435, 520.)* Darling v. Charleston Community Memorial Hospital (1965) established hospital liability for the actions of its employees. An 18-year-old football player fractured a leg, was treated in his local hospital over a 2-week period by a general practitioner without specialist consultation, subsequently developed complications, was transferred, and ultimately had a below-the-knee amputation. The physician settled out of court, but the case against the hospital continued with charges of negligence on a number of grounds, including failure to provide a sufficient number of trained nurses and failure of the nurses to bring the patient's condition to the attention of hospital officials so adequate consultation could be obtained. The hospital was found negligent and liable, thereby establishing the hospital's responsibility for the quality of the patient care administered in the institution. This also established the hospital's responsibility to monitor the credentials and competency of physicians.

The *Quinlan* case (1976) established that a patient's right to self-determination—and thus to decline medical treatment in certain situations—is protected by the right to privacy. The case involved a 21-year-old woman in a comatose vegetative state whose parents petitioned for the right to refuse treatment and turn off a respirator. The court reached its decision by balancing the state's interest in promoting the sanctity of life against the patient's privacy interest. The father was appointed legal guardian and in accordance with the findings of the hospital ethics committee, the respirator was turned off. Decisions regarding the withdrawal of life support remain very charged and controversial. Clear legal guidelines are still lacking for these decisions and individual decisions need to be made in each case with input from clinicians, ethicists, and often the courts.

Tarasoff v. *Regents of the University of California* (1976) confirmed the duty to warn. In the course of a psychotherapy session, a therapist was informed of a patient's intention to kill another person. The therapist failed to inform the victim of the patient's intentions, and the victim was subsequently murdered. The court held that the patient's right to privacy did not obviate the therapist's duty to warn possible victims in cases in which a therapist can *reasonably* determine that another person is at *foreseeable* risk. Performance of this duty may include notification of the police.

Roe v. *Wade* (1973) established the legal right to first- and second-trimester abortions in the United States and struck down almost all state laws forbidding such abortions. States can restrict third-trimester abortions, but not if the life or the health of the mother is in danger.

493–495. The answers are 493-c, 494-a, 495-d. (*Pozgar, 7/e, pp 59–66, 685.*) Abandonment is the unilateral termination of a doctor-patient relationship by the physician. It occurs when a physician terminates medical care prematurely (such as failing to follow up after an acute illness), fails to provide adequate cross-coverage, or refuses to see an established patient without notifying the patient and making arrangements to transfer care. The doctor-patient relationship may be ended by mutual consent of both parties, dismissal of the physician by the patient, absence of a requirement for continued medical care, or withdrawal of the physician with notification of the patient. This notification should be written and provide a reasonable transition period.

An assault is a threat to do harm. Battery involves touching another person in a socially unacceptable way without the person's consent. When informed consent is not obtained for medical procedures—diagnostic or therapeutic—battery is committed. The fact that the act may have improved the patient's health is legally irrelevant.

False imprisonment is the illegal confinement or restraint of a person or the illegal restraint of a person's liberty. A competent person who is not allowed to sign out against medical advice or who endures excessive use of physical restraints could sue for false imprisonment. Separate laws govern the involuntary hospitalization of the mentally ill.

496–498. The answers are 496-e, 497-a, 498-d. *(Beauchamp, 4/e, pp 54–55, 120–121, 227–237, 260–262, 498–499.)* Utilitarianism is the principle of doing the most good for the most people. It is useful in considering larger policy issues such as allocation of resources, but also applies to individual clinical decisions because, in situations where resources are limited, providing care for one person may well mean denying care for another. As a general rule, preventive care will produce greater utility per unit of medical care than will intensive care.

Autonomy is the competent person's moral right to select his or her own course of action; it is a cornerstone of medical ethics. The corresponding legal principle is self-determination. A competent person may refuse life-sustaining care and those wishes must be respected. Paternalistic behavior—that is, performing actions in a person's best interests against his or her wishes—is ethically and legally permissible only in very limited situations. The case of the AIDS patient's refusal of intubation illustrates a decision not to progress to further intervention in a fatal disease. It is not an example of "passive" euthanasia, the withdrawal of life-sustaining therapy; nor is it an example of "active" euthanasia, the administration of a lethal agent to end suffering.

A supererogatory act is one beyond the call of duty—one that is morally praiseworthy but cannot be required of a person. No one can claim a corresponding right to the performance of this act. Organ donation, stopping at roadside emergencies, or providing patients with a home phone number could all be acts of supererogation, albeit in decreasing order of importance.

Beneficence is the principle "to do good." Along with nonmaleficence, "to do no harm," it is one of the cornerstones of medical ethics.

499–500. The answers are 499-a, 500-d.   *(Pozgar, 7/e, pp 36, 66, 125.)* A tort is a civil wrong, other than a breach of contract. Written words of defamation are known as libel, while spoken words are known as slander. Antitrust laws protect against monopolies.

BIBLIOGRAPHY

AGENCY FOR HEALTH CARE POLICY AND RESEARCH (AHCPR): Smoking Cessation Clinical Practice Guidelines. Guideline 18, publication 96-0692. Rockville, MD, AHCPR, 1996.

AMERICAN ACADEMY OF PEDIATRICS: Policy statement: Recommendations for the prevention of pneumococcal infections, including the use of pneumococcal conjugate vaccine, pneumococcal polysaccharide vaccine and antibiotic prophylaxis. *Pediatrics* 106:362–366, 2000.

AMERICAN MEDICAL ASSOCIATION (AMA): Committee on Ethical and Judicial Affairs. 2000.

BEAUCHAMP TL, CHILDRESS JF: *Principles of Biomedical Ethics,* 4/e. New York, Oxford University Press, 1994.

CENTERS FOR DISEASE CONTROL AND PREVENTION (CDC): Case control study of HIV sero conversion in health care workers after percutaneous exposure to HIV-infected blood: France, United Kingdom, and United States. January 1988–August 1994. *MMWR* 40[RR-50]:929–933, 1995.

CENTERS FOR DISEASE CONTROL AND PREVENTION (CDC): Surveillance for waterborne-disease outbreaks: United States, 1993–1994. CDC Surveillance Summaries. *MMWR* 45(SS-1):1–34, 1996.

CENTERS FOR DISEASE CONTROL AND PREVENTION (CDC): Control and prevention of meningococcal disease and control and prevention of serogroup C meningococcal disease: Evaluation and management of suspected outbreaks. *MMWR* 46(RR-5):1–21, 1997.

CENTERS FOR DISEASE CONTROL AND PREVENTION (CDC): Guidelines for treatment of sexually transmitted diseases. *MMWR* 47(RR-1):1–111, 1998.

CENTERS FOR DISEASE CONTROL AND PREVENTION (CDC): Public health service guidelines for the management of health-care exposures to HIV and recommendation for post-exposure prophylaxis. *MMWR* 47(RR-7):1–28, 1998.

CENTERS FOR DISEASE CONTROL AND PREVENTION (CDC): Measles, mumps, rubella vaccine use and strategies in the USA for elimination of congenital rubella syndrome and control of mumps—Recommendations from ACIP. *MMWR* 47(RR-8):1–57, 1998.

CENTERS FOR DISEASE CONTROL AND PREVENTION (CDC): Recommendations for prevention and control of hepatitis C virus (HCV) infection and HCV-related chronic disease. *MMWR* 47(RR-19):1–39, 1998.

CENTERS FOR DISEASE CONTROL AND PREVENTION (CDC): Prevention and treatment of tuberculosis among patients infected with HIV: Principles of therapy and revised recommendations. *MMWR* 47(RR-20):1–58, 1998.

CENTERS FOR DISEASE CONTROL AND PREVENTION (CDC): Guidelines for vaccinating pregnant women—Recommendations from ACIP. DHHS, 1998.

CENTERS FOR DISEASE CONTROL AND PREVENTION (CDC): *STD surveillance report—US 1998.* Division of STD Prevention, 1999.

CENTERS FOR DISEASE CONTROL AND PREVENTION (CDC): Withdrawal of rotavirus vaccine recommendation. *JAMA* 282:2113–2114, 1999.

CENTERS FOR DISEASE CONTROL AND PREVENTION (CDC): Achievements in public health, 1990–1999: Healthier mothers and babies. *MMWR* 48:849–858, 1999.

CENTERS FOR DISEASE CONTROL AND PREVENTION (CDC): Human rabies prevention—United States, 1999: Recommendations of the Advisory Committee on Immunization Practices (ACIP). *MMWR* 48(RR-1):1–21, 1999.

CENTERS FOR DISEASE CONTROL AND PREVENTION (CDC): Prevention and control of influenza—Recommendations from ACIP. *MMWR* 48(RR-4): 1–28, 1999.

CENTERS FOR DISEASE CONTROL AND PREVENTION (CDC): Prevention of varicella. Update recommendations from ACIP. *MMWR* 48(RR-6):1–5, 1999.

CENTERS FOR DISEASE CONTROL AND PREVENTION (CDC): Recommendations for the use of Lyme vaccine—Recommendations from the ACIP. *MMWR* 48(RR-7):1–25, 1999.

CENTERS FOR DISEASE CONTROL AND PREVENTION (CDC): Vaccine-preventable diseases: Improving vaccination coverage in children, adolescents and adults. *MMWR* 48(RR-8):1–15, 1999.

CENTERS FOR DISEASE CONTROL AND PREVENTION (CDC): Prevention of hepatitis A through active or passive immunization—Recommendations from ACIP. *MMWR* 48(RR-12):1–37, 1999.

CENTERS FOR DISEASE CONTROL AND PREVENTION (CDC): Outbreak of West Nile-like viral encephalitis—New York, 1999. *MMWR* 48(RR-39): 871–874, 1999.

CENTERS FOR DISEASE CONTROL AND PREVENTION (CDC): Abortion surveillance—United States, 1996. *MMWR* 48(SS-5):1–44, 1999.

CENTERS FOR DISEASE CONTROL AND PREVENTION (CDC): Monitoring hospital-acquired infections to promote patient safety—United States, 1990–1999. *MMWR* 49(RR-8):149–153, 2000.

CHIN J: *Control of Communicable Diseases Manual, 17/e.* Washington, DC, American Public Health Association, 2000.

CHRISTOFFEL T, GALLAGHER SS: *Injury Prevention and Public Health.* Gaithersburg, MD, Aspen Publication, 1999.

ENGLISH DC: *Bioethics: A Clinical Guide for Medical Students.* New York, Norton and Norton, 1994.

THE EUROPEAN MODE OF DELIVERY COLLABORATION. Elective caesarian-section versus vaginal delivery in prevention of vertical HIV-1 transmission: A randomized clinical trial. *Lancet* 353:1035–1039, 1999.

FAUCI AS, BRAUNWALD E, ISSELBACHER KJ, ET AL: *Harrison's Principles of Internal Medicine, 14/e.* New York, McGraw-Hill, 1998.

FAUCI AS, BRAUNWALD E, ISSELBACHER KJ, ET AL: *Harrison's Principles of Internal Medicine, Companion Handbook, 14/e.* New York, McGraw-Hill, 1998.

GABEL J: Ten ways HMOs have changed during the 1990s. *Health Affairs* 16:134–144, 1997.

GREENBERG RS, DANIELS SR, FLANDERS WD, ET AL: *Medical Epidemiology, 2/e,* East Norwalk, CT, Appleton & Lange, 1996.

HENNEKENS CH, BURING JE: *Epidemiology in Medicine.* Boston, Little, Brown, 1987.

HOLMES KK, SPARLING PF, MARDH PE ET AL. (EDS): *Sexually Transmitted Diseases, 3/e.* New York, McGraw-Hill, 1999.

INGELFINGER J, MOSTELLER F, THIBODEAU LA, WARE JH: *Biostatistics in Clinical Medicine, 3/e.* New York, McGraw-Hill, 1994.

JEKEL JF: *Epidemiology, Biostatistics and Preventive Medicine.* Philadelphia, W. B. Saunders Company, 1996.

KOZARSKY PE: Prevention of common travel ailments. *Infectious Disease Clinics of North America* 12:305–323, 1998.

LADOU J: *Occupational and Environmental Medicine, 2/e.* Stamford, CT, Appleton & Lange, 1997.

MASSACHUSETTS DEPARTMENT OF PUBLIC HEALTH (MDPH): *Foodborne Illness Investigation and Control, Reference Manual.* Boston, Division of Epidemiology and Immunization, Division of Food and Drug, Division of Diagnostic Laboratories, 1999.

THE MEDICAL FOUNDATION. *Where There's Smoke, There's Disease: Reducing the Effects of Environmental Tobacco Smoke in Massachusetts.* Boston, The Medical Foundation, 1999.

NAWAZ H, KATZ DL: American College of Preventive Medicine policy statement: Perimenopausal and postmenopausal hormone replacement therapy. *Am J Prev Med* 17:250–254, 1999.

NATIONAL VACCINE ADVISORY COMMITTEE (NVAC): Strategies to sustain success in childhood immunizations. Consensus statement. *JAMA* 282: 363–370, 1999.

PARAN TV: The physician's role in smoking cessation. *J Respiratory Diseases* 19(5)S6-12, 1998.

PAGANO M, GAUVREAU K: *Principles of Biostatistics.* Belmont, CA, Duxbury, 1993.

POTTERAT JJ, ROTHENBERG RB, MUTH JB, ET AL: Invoking, monitoring, and relinquishing a public health power. *Sex Trans Dis* 26:345–349, 1999.

POZGAR GD: *Legal Aspects of Health Care Administration, 7/e.* Rockville, MD, Aspen, 1998.

RICHARDS EP, RATHBURN KC: The role of police power in 21st century public health. *Sex Trans Dis* 26:350–357, 1999.

ROSNER B: *Fundamentals of Biostatistics, 5/e.* Pacific Grove, CA, Duxbury, 2000.

RYAN ET, KAIN KC. Primary care: Health advice and immunizations for travelers. *NEJM* 342:1716–1725, 2000.

SCHNEIDER MJ: *Introduction to Public Health.* Gaithersburg, MD, Aspen Publications, 2000.

SCUTCHFIELD FD, KECK CW: *Principles of Public Health Practice.* Albany, NY, Delmar Publishers, 1997.

US DEPARTMENT OF HEALTH AND HUMAN SERVICE (USDHHS): *Healthy people 2010: Understanding and improving health.* Washington DC, USDHHS, 1999.

US DEPARTMENT OF HEALTH AND HUMAN SERVICES (USDHHS), PUBLIC HEALTH SERVICES (PHS), CDC. *STD surveillance 1998.* Atlanta, GA, USDHHS, PHS, 1999.

US PREVENTIVE SERVICES (USPS) TASK FORCE. *Guide to Clinical Preventive Services, 2/e.* Baltimore, MD, Williams & Wilkins, 1996.

WALLACE RB, DOEBBELING BN, LAST JM ET AL: *Maxcy-Rosenau-Last Public Health and Preventive Medicine, 14/e.* Stamford, CT, Appleton & Lange, 1998.

Notes

Notes

Notes

Notes

Notes

Notes